Handbook of
Clinical Neurology

Handbook of Clinical Neurology

V Natarajan MD DM (Neurology) FRCP (Edinburgh) FAAN FIAN FIMSA
Former Professor and Head
Madras Institute of Neurology
Madras Medical College, Chennai
Professor Emeritus
The Tamil Nadu Dr MGR Medical University
Chennai, Tamil Nadu, India

K Mugundhan MD DM (Neurology) FRCP (Edinburgh) FRCP (London)
FRCP (Glasgow) FRCP (Ireland) FACP FICP FIMSA
Professor and Head
Department of Neurology
Stanley Medical College
Chennai, Tamil Nadu, India

Forewords
A Muruganathan
R Rajasekar

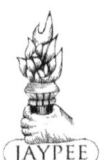

JAYPEE BROTHERS MEDICAL PUBLISHERS
The Health Sciences Publisher
New Delhi | London

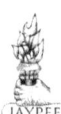 **Jaypee Brothers Medical Publishers (P) Ltd**

Headquarters
EMCA House
23/23-B, Ansari Road, Daryaganj
New Delhi 110 002, India
Landline: +91-11-23272143, +91-11-23272703
+91-11-23282021, +91-11-23245672
E-mail: jaypee@jaypeebrothers.com

Corporate Office
Jaypee Brothers Medical Publishers (P) Ltd.
4838/24, Ansari Road, Daryaganj
New Delhi 110 002, India
Phone: +91-11-43574357
Fax: +91-11-43574314
E-mail: jaypee@jaypeebrothers.com

Overseas Office
JP Medical Ltd.
83, Victoria Street, London
SW1H 0HW (UK)
Phone: +44-20 3170 8910
Fax: +44(0)20 3008 6180
E-mail: info@jpmedpub.com

Website: www.jaypeebrothers.com
Website: www.jaypeedigital.com

© 2024, Jaypee Brothers Medical Publishers

The views and opinions expressed in this book are solely those of the original contributor(s)/author(s) and do not necessarily represent those of editor(s) or publisher of the book.

All rights reserved. No part of this publication may be reproduced, stored or transmitted in any form or by any means, electronic, mechanical, photocopying, recording or otherwise, without the prior permission in writing of the publishers.

All brand names and product names used in this book are trade names, service marks, trademarks or registered trademarks of their respective owners. The publisher is not associated with any product or vendor mentioned in this book.

Medical knowledge and practice change constantly. This book is designed to provide accurate, authoritative information about the subject matter in question. However, readers are advised to check the most current information available on procedures included and check information from the manufacturer of each product to be administered, to verify the recommended dose, formula, method and duration of administration, adverse effects and contraindications. It is the responsibility of the practitioner to take all appropriate safety precautions. Neither the publisher nor the author(s)/editor(s) assume any liability for any injury and/or damage to persons or property arising from or related to use of material in this book.

This book is sold on the understanding that the publisher is not engaged in providing professional medical services. If such advice or services are required, the services of a competent medical professional should be sought.

Every effort has been made where necessary to contact holders of copyright to obtain permission to reproduce copyright material. If any have been inadvertently overlooked, the publisher will be pleased to make the necessary arrangements at the first opportunity.

Inquiries for bulk sales may be solicited at: jaypee@jaypeebrothers.com

Handbook of Clinical Neurology / V Natarajan, K Mugundhan
First Edition: **2024**
ISBN: 978-93-5696-369-6

Foreword

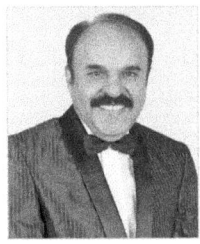

A Muruganathan MD FICP FRCP (Glasgow & London)
FRCP (Ireland) (Hon) FACP (USA) FPCP (Philippines)
Imm. Past Governor, American College of Physicians, India Chapter
Dean, Indian College of Physicians (ICP), 2016–2017
President, Hypertension Society of India (HSI), 2015–2016
President, Association of Physicians of India (API), 2013–2014

I am pleased to write the foreword for this interesting book "*Handbook of Clinical Neurology*" written by my good friends Professor Dr V Natarajan and coauthored by Professor Dr K Mugundhan.

A good general physician is a jack of all trades and he should know how to diagnose a disease and treat it properly. I went through the contents of the book. The authors have discussed the subject in two sections: Sections 1 and 2. Section 1 includes a practical approach to neurological symptoms such as headache, dizziness, seizures, limb weakness, speech abnormality, and visual symptoms. These symptoms are present in many systemic disorders. A physician must approach a patient by taking a detailed clinical history and possess a good knowledge about clinical examination. This would help him to arrive at a diagnosis and manage it properly. This book gives the practicing physician useful tips for managing the patient. In Section 2, the authors discuss an overview of common neurological disorders such as stroke, autoimmune neurologic disorders, movement disorders, infection of the nervous system, and the importance of dementia.

All relevant points for the above diseases and the best method for the practical approach are nicely explained in this book. I hope this book finds a place in every physician's clinical chamber. I congratulate the authors for bringing out such a useful book.

A Muruganathan

Foreword

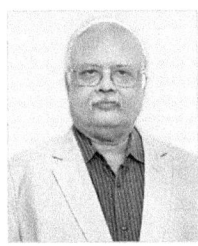

R Rajasekar MD FICP FACP (USA)
FRCP (Glasgow, Ireland, London, and Edinburgh)
Senior Consultant Physician and Diabetologist
Chairman, RR Charitable and Educational Trust
Heart and Diabetes Therapy Centre
Diabetes Training Centre for Doctors
Kumbakonam, Tamil Nadu, India

It is my pride to write a foreword for the book titled *"Handbook of Clinical Neurology"*. I eulogize the authors, Professors Drs V Natarajan and K Mugundhan for having written this book in a pellucid manner. I am happy to say that Dr V Natarajan has been instrumental in creating many neurologists by his masterly teaching and guidance.

Their approach is very practical and crystal clear. I am sure it will be of great benefit to all postgraduates and medical practitioners. The authors' commitment to writing this book is very much appreciable.

R Rajasekar

Preface

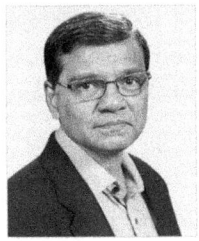

V Natarajan MD DM (Neurology)
FRCP (Edinburgh) FAAN FIAN FIMSA

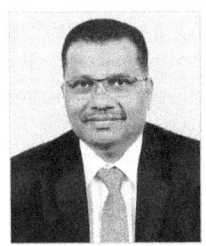

K Mugundhan MD DM (Neurology)
FRCP (Edinburgh) FRCP (London) FRCP (Glasgow) FRCP (Ireland) FACP FICP FIMSA

In today's practice, it is imperative that a practicing physician is conversant with the common problems in every subspecialty of medicine. This has become all the more important now, as technology-provided expertise is available to every practicing physician that helps in the diagnosis and management of the subspecialty-related problems. Patients with neurological symptoms getting admitted to hospitals directly under the practicing physician has become common, and an opinion is thereafter obtained from the neurologist, following which the admitting physician continues with the management of the patient. In this scenario, an understanding of the patient's symptoms and his causes would enhance the physician's ability to manage the patient's problem confidently.

This handbook aims to fulfill this purpose, by providing essential information on how to approach each of the common neurologic symptoms faced in practice by the physician. An analytic approach to the symptoms is adopted which would help the physician to formulate a differential diagnosis and investigate appropriately and manage.

The style of presentation in this handbook is essentially practice oriented and stems from the experience of the first author gathered over 40 years of neurologic practice. The co-author Dr K Mugundhan has added his observations and experience bolstered with appropriate charts, diagrams, and pictures, to enhance the ease of assimilation of the information provided.

Preface

We wish to emphasize that this handbook has been written in a simple, easy-to-read style to enhance your understanding and enable efficient, confident handling of the neurological problems. This handbook does not purport to be a textbook by any means, and the readers are requested to refer to textbooks of neurology, to get additional information whenever required. However, we have ensured that the section of overview of common neurological disorders includes relevant information on the disorders discussed in the section.

V Natarajan
K Mugundhan

Acknowledgments

We are extremely grateful to Dr A Muruganathan for his kind words in the foreword.

We would like to thank our friend and motivator Dr R Rajasekar for his constant encouragement in bringing out this handbook and also his kind words in the foreword.

We are deeply indebted to our teachers Professors K Jagannathan, G Arjundas, K Srinivas, Zaheer Ahmed Sayeed, and CU Velmurugendran, all former professors at the Institute of Neurology, Chennai, whose inspiration and guidance have been the biggest strength and source of knowledge to the first author.

We are grateful to our colleagues Drs PR Sowmini and M Sathish Kumar, Assistant Professors of Neurology, Stanley Medical College, Chennai, Tamil Nadu, India, for their contribution with suggestions and help in corrections.

We would like to thank all our patients who were the true sources of the material for this book.

We would also like to extend our gratitude to our family members for their patience and support.

Thanks are due to the publishers for encouraging and putting up with us with repeated corrections.

Contents

Section 1: Practical Approach to Neurological Symptoms

Chapter 1: Headache 3

Chapter 2: Dizziness and Vertigo 10

Chapter 3: Seizures 19

Chapter 4: Limb Weakness 25

Chapter 5: Speech Abnormalities 39

Chapter 6: Visual Symptoms 42

Chapter 7: Assessment of Higher Functions 48

Chapter 8: Assessment of Sensorium 62

Section 2: Overview of Common Neurologic Disorders

Chapter 9: Stroke 69

Chapter 10: Autoimmune Neurologic Disorders 82

Chapter 11: Movement Disorders 94

Chapter 12: Infections of the Nervous System 116

Chapter 13: Dementia 127

Index 143

SECTION 1

Practical Approach to Neurological Symptoms

CHAPTER 1: Headache

CHAPTER 2: Dizziness and Vertigo

CHAPTER 3: Seizures

CHAPTER 4: Limb Weakness

CHAPTER 5: Speech Abnormalities

CHAPTER 6: Visual Symptoms

CHAPTER 7: Assessment of Higher Functions

CHAPTER 8: Assessment of Sensorium

CHAPTER 1

Headache

INTRODUCTION

Headache is one of the most common neurological symptoms.
- The objective of the physician would be to differentiate the sinister causes of headache from the benign ones.
- An understanding (knowledge) of the benign types of headaches would help to differentiate them from the more serious causes.
- The benign headaches are grouped under primary headaches, meaning that there are no underlying causes triggering these headaches.
- The headaches which have an underlying cause are considered as secondary headaches and it is these headaches which the physician needs to be wary of and identify.

The following are the common primary headache disorders:
- Migraine
- Tension-type headache (TTH)
- Trigeminal autonomic cephalgias (TAC)

MIGRAINE

Migraine is arguably the most common type of primary headache vying with TTH for the top spot. Quite often, migraine and TTHs occur in the same person, at different times, making the detection of the frequency of each of these difficult.

According to a study conducted by the National Institute of Mental Health and Neurosciences (NIMHANs), one in five persons in the population of South India could have migraine. The diagnosis of migraine is essentially based on the history of the patient. The characteristics of migraine headaches are as follows:
- They are episodic and recurrent and can occur at different sites over the head (temporal, ocular, frontal, temporoparietal, occipital, and nuchal).
- They are usually unilateral and side shifting but can also be bilateral **(Fig. 1)**.
- They are usually throbbing in nature and last from hours to a day and at times up to 3 days.
- Nausea, vomiting, intolerance to sound (phonophobia), intolerance to bright light (photophobia), and intolerance to strong smell (osmophobia) are characteristic features with only one of these, phonophobia or photophobia, being associated with TTHs.
- There are several triggers to migraine headache-like exposure to sunlight, inadequate sleep, stress, perimenstrual period, long distance travel, head bath, hunger, and seasonal changes.

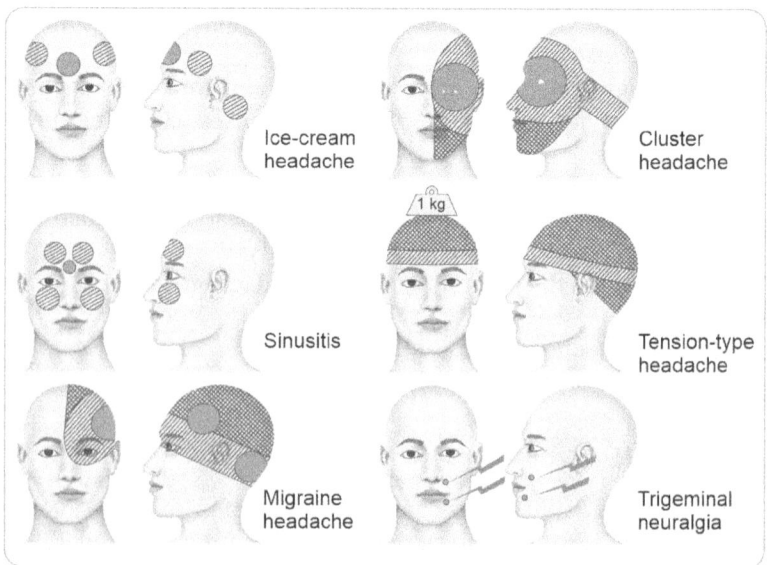

FIG. 1: Sites of various types of headache.

Invariably, these headaches run in the family and most often one of the parents, especially the mother, or siblings would be having such episodic headache.

If the majority of the above-described features can be obtained on elicitation of the history, and if the patient does not have abnormal signs on neurological examination, the diagnosis of migraine is reasonably certain and no imaging will be required, unless the person develops new symptoms or shows signs on examination during follow-up. Migraine can occur in children as well, though usually, the onset is in the 2nd or 3rd decade. Trauma can trigger migraine headaches at a later age.

Migraine is of two types:
1. Migraine without aura, which is the more common type of migraine
2. Migraine with aura, where there is an aura preceding the headache or associated at onset, which is relatively uncommon

Visual, sensory, or motor symptoms are the various forms of auras. Visual aura is the most frequent of the auras and can take the form of dazzling lights, lightning-like streaks, zigzag lines going across, paracentral scotomas, expanding toward the periphery and becoming colored (scintillating).

Sensory aura is not as common as visual aura but is often not recognized and has to be asked for. It is most often described as an abnormal sensory feel or numbness in the upper limbs and sometimes in the chest as well. Rarely, dysphasia can occur as a speech aura.

A number of drugs can be tried as prophylaxis for reducing the frequency of migraine episodes. Propranolol, amitriptyline, valproic acid, topiramate, and flunarizine can be tried in acceptable doses, and the choice depends on the which comorbidity the person has.

TENSION-TYPE HEADACHE

Tension-type headache is the other common type of headache. This is a more chronic and longer-lasting headache, which is usually felt over the vertex or the entire head, and does not shift sites and is seldom unilateral.

These headaches are not associated with nausea or vomiting and do not have specific triggers, though these could be associated with either photo- or phonophobia but usually not both.

The pain is felt as though a weight is placed over the head or a tight band is tied tight across the head. As mentioned earlier, TTH and migraine can occur at different periods in the same individual.

These episodes can be treated with nonsteroidal anti-inflammatory drugs (NSAIDs) or paracetamol for relief, and recurrent or chronic occurrence can be reduced with tricyclic antidepressants given on a short-term basis as required, depending on the frequency of occurrence.

TRIGEMINAL AUTONOMIC CEPHALGIAS

Cluster Headache

A cluster headache is a specific type of headache having unique characteristics:
- The episodes are characterized by severe, nonfluctuating, nonpulsatile, periorbital and/or temporal pain, always occurring on the same side and reaching crescendo within 10 minutes.
- Episodes last from 30 minutes to 2 hours and occur almost daily for periods ranging from 2 to 4 weeks with a pain-free interval in between, lasting from 3 months to a year, showing a periodicity.
- The patient is restless and keeps pacing during the headache, which is a key feature.
- Another characteristic feature is the occurrence of autonomic features such as lacrimation, redness of the eye, and congestion of the nose, all on the ipsilateral side of the headache due to sudden release of hypothalamus-driven serotonin and histamine.
- It is more common in men in the 3rd to 5th decade and is related to smoking and taking alcohol.

Acute treatment includes 100% O_2 through a nasal mask which is practically difficult to administer. Sumatriptan 6 mg subcutaneously (SC) or as nasal spray and dihydroergotamine 0.5–1 mg SC or intramuscularly (IM) are other medications used for relief.

Preventive Treatment

The following medications can be tried for preventive treatment:
- Oral steroids, which are also effective in aborting the acute episodes, 50–60 mg/day and tapered off over 3–6 weeks
- Verapamil— 40–200 mg/day

- Lithium—600-900 mg/day, but this is a little difficult to monitor and maintain over a long-term basis

Other types of TACs are more rare and include the following.

Paroxysmal Hemicrania
- The pain is usually periorbital in location but can be more extensive. It remains unilateral and is associated with the autonomic symptoms described under cluster headache.
- Pain is shorter lasting for a maximum period of 30 minutes unlike cluster headache which lasts longer and is exquisitely responsive to indomethacin, which is a characteristic diagnostic feature.

SUNCT
Short-lasting unilateral neuralgiform headache attacks with conjunctival injection and tearing (SUNCT) is very rare, manifesting as brief episodes lasting for a few seconds and as multiple attacks in a day, associated with lacrimation and redness of the eye.

Treatment
Lamotrigine—100-300 mg/day—is recommended.

Secondary Headaches
A secondary headache is likely when neurological examination is abnormal with the presence of papilledema, cranial nerve palsies, or pyramidal signs in the form of weakness or abnormal reflexes considered the "Red Flag Signs".
- Acute or sudden onset of headache or the first or worst ever headache
- A new-onset or late-onset headache
- Progressive or worsening headache
- Headache with neurological symptoms and signs, as mentioned above

It is also likely that the history of headache is not classical as that of the primary headaches described above and is atypical, in which case the patient will have to be evaluated for an underlying cause, with the following investigations as appropriate:
- *Imaging*: To identify space-occupying lesions such as tumors, abscess, and granulomas; vascular events such as intracranial hemorrhage; and cerebral venous sinus thrombosis

- *Cerebrospinal fluid (CSF) study*: For detection of infections and subarachnoid hemorrhage
- *Erythrocyte sedimentation rate (ESR) and C reactive protein (CRP)*: To identify temporal arteritis (TA) as a possible cause of the headache
- Ophthalmic and an ear, nose and throat specialists (ENT) check for excluding ophthalmic and ENT causes of the headache

Temporal Arteritis

Temporal arteritis is an inflammatory disease involving the temporal artery. It is unilateral, occurring in elderly women, with pain being aggravated on jaw movement and is usually associated with weight loss, with or without fever, and with scalp tenderness as characteristic features. Increased ESR and CRP, and remission with oral steroids, are further clues to the diagnosis. Temporal artery biopsy is considered diagnostic and needs to be done to establish the diagnosis, if in doubt.

Idiopathic Intracranial Hypertension

The clinical features of increased intracranial tension (ICT) are symptoms such as headache, vomiting, transient obscuration of vision, and presence of papilledema on examination. There should be no structural abnormality or venous sinus thrombosis on imaging, and the CSF should reveal increased opening pressure to confirm the diagnosis.

Magnetic resonance imaging (MRI) might show perioptic sheath widening, partial empty sella, and flattening of the posterior part of the globe with no evidence of cerebral venous sinus thrombosis.

Treatment consists of repeated lumbar punctures (LP) and letting out of CSF, and acetazolamide orally as 250 mg tablets 4 times a day (1 gm/day). Optic nerve sheath fenestration or ventriculoperitoneal shunt is done when vision is threatened in spite of the above measures, though optic nerve sheath fenestration is not widely practiced.

Spontaneous Intracranial Hypotension

Spontaneous intracranial hypotension (SICH) is a condition wherein there is reduced pressure within the intracranial cavity due to the leak of CSF following LP or due to an acquired leak in the dura mater, which gives rise to the headache.

It is diagnosed by MRI findings of the sagging of posterior fossa contents, pachymeningeal contrast enhancement, a history of headache occurring in the erect position (sitting or standing), and reducing on lying supine.

This condition is treated with increased fluid administration and assumption of supine posture. If it is persistent, a blood patch at the site of leak in the dura mater may be required.

Thunderclap Headache

The term "thunderclap headache" is applied to a headache which is very intense and reaches its peak within seconds (<30 seconds) and lasts from an hour to days.

Though this could be a primary headache, an underlying vascular cause has to be excluded such as reversible cerebral vasoconstriction syndrome (RCVS), subarachnoid hemorrhage, cerebral venous sinus thrombosis, intracerebral hemorrhage, cerebellar hemorrhage, pituitary apoplexy, accentuated hypertension, aneurysmal bleed, arteriovenous malformation (AVM) bleeds, cerebral amyloid angiopathy, and arterial dissection, and hence imaging would be the investigation of choice in this scenario.

Medication-overuse Headache

In this condition, the headache occurs almost daily and the person becomes dependent on an analgesic to get rid of the headache and this becomes a vicious cycle. Medication-overuse headache (MOH) needs to be differentiated from chronic daily headache, which is considered to be a form of transformed migraine. Because of analgesic dependence, the patient feels the presence of headache if the analgesic is not taken. Both chronic daily headache and MOH need to be treated with preventive medications, the only difference being that patients with MOHs should be dissuaded from taking analgesics.

Migralepsy

Persons with migraine can exhibit loss of consciousness and at times can have even clonic movements at the peak of their headaches. This condition has been termed migralepsy, when both headache and seizures occur together, with the headache occurring earlier, followed by the seizures during the episode.

CHAPTER 2

Dizziness and Vertigo

INTRODUCTION

Diagnosing dizziness can be difficult, and it can have serious consequences if dangerous causes, including stroke, are overlooked. Specific findings are frequently discernible with knowledge of the neuro-otological bedside examination.

DIZZINESS

Dizziness is a common symptom faced by all physicians in their clinical practice. The term dizziness includes a host of symptoms signifying vertigo, light headedness, mental confusion, generalized weakness, disorientation, presyncope, and postural instability.

Recognizing the dizziness pattern narrows down the differential diagnosis. The recurrent and troublesome type of dizziness is the vertigo. Vertigo is a sense of rotation of the head (subjective vertigo) or rotation of the environment (objective vertigo).

Vertigo can be brief, lasting a few seconds, a few minutes, or a few hours, and can be recurrent. Occasionally, vertigo can be prolonged lasting for a few days but such occurrences are usually infrequent. Most of the recurrent vertigo episodes are benign. Acute onset of protracted vertigo with nausea and vomiting indicates vestibular neuritis and when associated with hearing loss, it is indicative of labyrinthitis. Vertigo associated with vegetative symptoms such as recurrent vomiting, sweating, and palpitations is usually indicative of a peripheral vestibular system involvement. Unilateral horizontal or upbeat torsional nystagmus confirms a peripheral vestibular disturbance.

The head impulse test (HIT) is a useful test to assess the vestibular system. To do this test, the patient is asked to fix his vision steadfast on the examiner's nose, and the examiner turns the head of the subject 20° briskly to either side, taking care to avoid injury to the neck. The test is considered positive if the subject's eyes move passively in the direction of the head movement with a corrective saccade bringing it back to the fixation point. The side to which the eyes move with the head turn is considered to be the damaged side. In the rare event of a bilateral vestibulopathy, the test is positive on both sides. The VEMP (vestibular evoked myogenic potential) study if available, could further corroborate the involvement of the peripheral vestibular system. This test is also called the head-thrust test (HTT) **(Figs. 1A and B)**.

COMMON TYPES OF VERTIGO

Benign Paroxysmal Positional Vertigo

When the patient rolls over, lies down, or turns in bed, the semicircular canals are stimulated, causing calcium-containing otolith debris in the semicircular canals to shift. The Dix–Hallpike maneuver is a useful test which is sensitive and specific for benign paroxysmal positional vertigo (BPPV). The patient is brought to the edge of the bed with the head hanging down and the head is turned to right and left and observed for the occurrence of nystagmus. The nystagmus occurs according to the position of the head and is paroxysmal and this is important, as nonparoxysmal occurrence would indicate a central cause. The particular head position would need to be held for at least 10 seconds in order to elicit the nystagmus since the commencement of the nystagmus would be delayed. With repeated testing, this nystagmus's severity lessens and it is fatigable. When the posterior canal is affected, which is the most common variety, the nystagmus would be upbeat and torsional with the upper half of the eyes

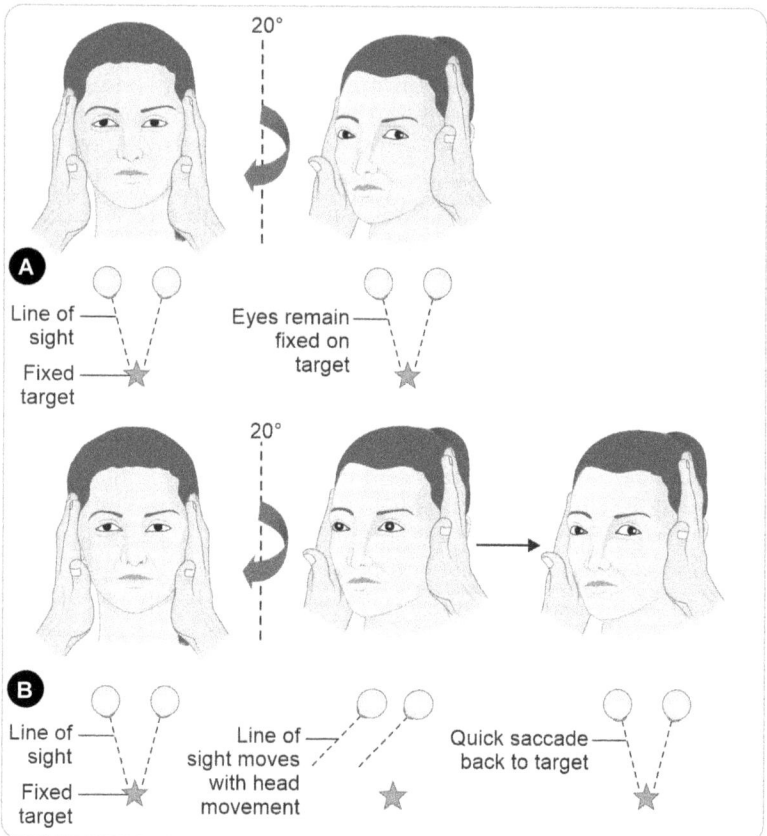

FIGS. 1A AND B: Head-thrust test. A simple test for vestibular function that may be performed at the bedside is the head-thrust test. The vestibulo-ocular reflex (VOR) is put to the test in this maneuver. The patient is seated in front of the examiner, who maintains a steady midline grasp on the patient's head. The patient is told to keep looking at the examiner's nose. The examiner next abruptly tilts the patient's head 10–15° to one side and checks the patient's ability to maintain eye contact with his or her nose. The peripheral vestibular system is presumed to be in good working order if the patient's eyes remain fixed on the examiner's nose (i.e., there is no corrective saccade) (A). However, if the patient's eyes move with the head (B) and then the patient voluntarily moves their eyes back to the examiner's nose (i.e., a corrective saccade), this suggests a peripheral vestibular system lesion rather than a central nervous system (CNS) lesion.

beating toward the ground. The nystagmus is primarily horizontal when the horizontal canal is implicated, and it is downbeat when the anterior canal, which is the least common, is involved **(Figs. 2A and B)**.

CHAPTER 2: Dizziness and Vertigo

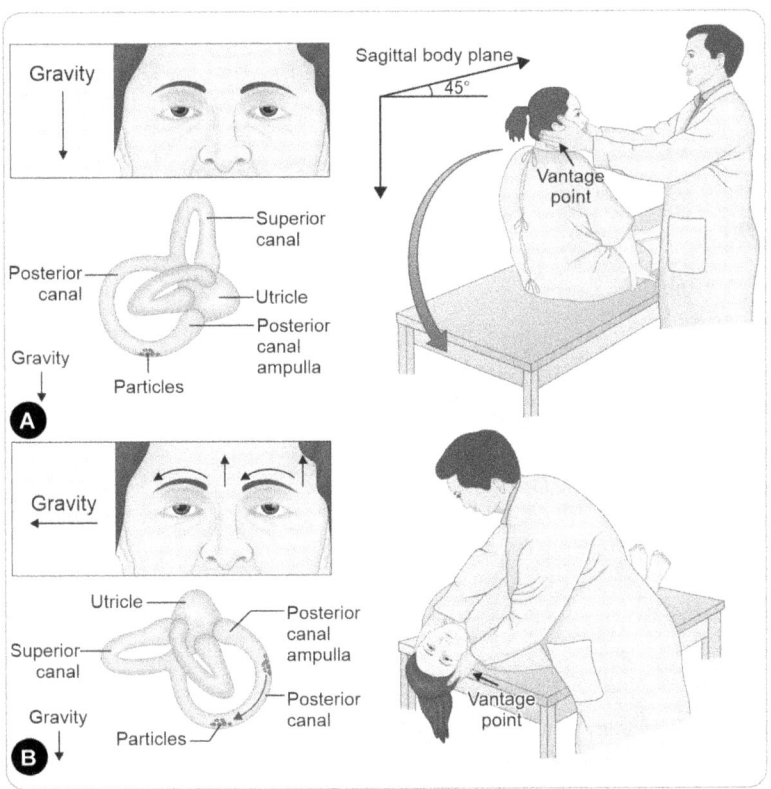

FIGS. 2A AND B: Dix–Hallpike maneuver: (A) To line the right posterior semicircular canal with the body's sagittal plane, the examiner adopts a 45° right angle while standing at the patient's head. (B) The examiner shifts the patient, whose eyes are open, from the seated to the supine position with the right ear down. Then, the examiner extends the patient's neck slightly to make the chin point upward. If nystagmus and vertigo are present, it is important to take note of their latency, duration, and direction.

The Epley maneuver which repositions the particles is usually effective in relief of BPPV **(Fig. 3)**.

Vestibular Migraine or Migrainous Vertigo

The other common cause of recurrent vertigo is vestibular migraine, which is being increasingly recognized now, though thought to be rare earlier.

Vestibular migraine could be an association of vertigo and headache occurring together or vertigo occurring with associated

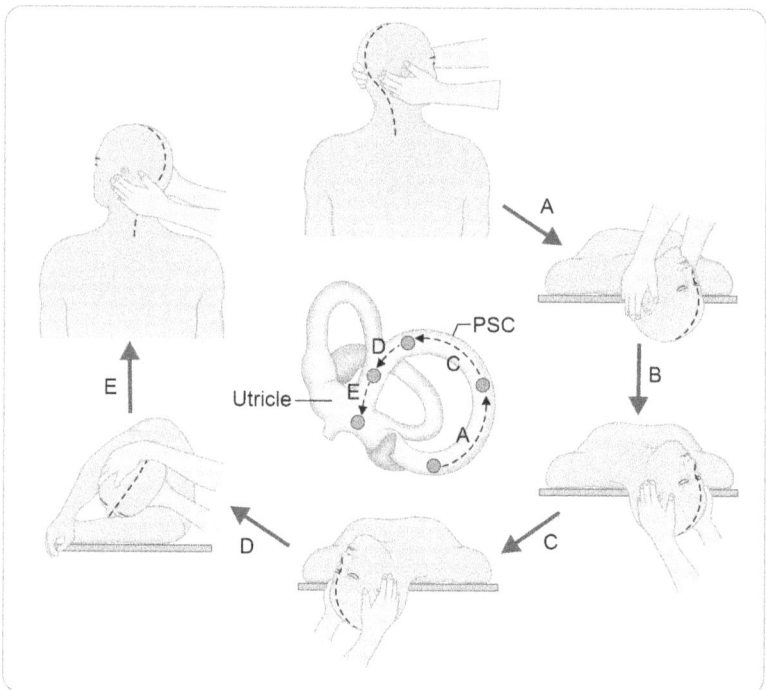

FIG. 3: The Epley's maneuver used to treat right ear benign paroxysmal positional vertigo. In order to treat the left ear, the procedure might be reversed. The position of the debris as it travels through the posterior semicircular canal (PSC) and into the utricle (UT) are depicted in the labyrinth drawing in the center. A—the patient is sat upright and is looking at the right-side-standing examiner. B—the patient is quickly transferred into the correct head-hanging position for the Dix–Hallpike test. The patient remains in this position until the nystagmus stops. Examiner positions hands as depicted before moving to the head of the table. C—the right ear is raised as the patient's head is quickly turned to the left. For 30 seconds, this position is held. D—the patient rolls over onto his left side as the examiner quickly turns his head to the left till the nose is pointed at the ground. The next 30 seconds are spent holding the head this position. E—the patient is then swiftly raised a sitting posture, the head facing left this time, the entire procedure should be repeated till there is no nystagmus. In order to prevent the debris from reentering the posterior canal after the maneuver, the patient should be advised to refrain from head-hanging positions.

features like photophobia and being triggered by the triggers of migraine headache which enhances the diagnosis. The vertigo lasts for minutes to an hour with fluctuating intensity and could be associated with a feel of generalized weakness.

Vestibular Neuritis

Acute onset of vertigo which is severe, and is associated with recurrent nausea and vomiting from onset, and reduces thereafter and lasts for days, should prompt the diagnosis of acute vestibular neuritis. This occurs usually due to a viral infection or reactivation of latent viruses in the vestibular nerve ganglion.

Spontaneous, unidirectional nystagmus beating away from the involved ear and associated with an abnormal gait on the first day, with the patient, and tending to fall toward the side of the lesion are features, which confirm this diagnosis. If a new ipsilateral hearing loss is also associated with the above, the condition is called labyrinthitis. Early corticosteroid therapy would hasten the recovery, along with a short use of vestibular sedatives.

Transient Ischemic Attack

It is one of the important differential diagnosis of a brief episode of dizziness or vertigo but is never an isolated symptom and it is usually associated with visual disturbance, confusion, or altered sensorium albeit brief.

HINTS (*H*ead, *I*mpulse, *N*ystagmus, *T*est of *S*kew battery) helps to distinguish a central from a peripheral vertigo. Signs of long tracts (motor or sensory) and cranial nerves (neighborhood signs) involvement indicate a central cause.

The nonvestibular system dysfunction cause of dizziness would include:
- Global cerebral ischemia which causes lightheadedness which improves with the patient lying down. When dizziness is associated with blurred vision and tachycardia on standing, global cerebral ischemia should be suspected which leads to presyncope or syncope.
- Other differential diagnosis would be dysautonomia and cardiac arrhythmias. The causes of dysautonomia would include B12 deficiency, diabetes mellitus, peripheral neuropathy (PN), and neurodegenerative brain disorders.

Dizziness and Anxiety

Anxiety can manifest as dizziness and chronic vestibular dysfunction can also cause anxiety. Occasionally, anxiety is due to dizziness caused by an independent dysautonomia as an associated feature.

Dysautonomia can cause dizziness and anxiety.

Sensitivity to movement of objects is a feature of dizziness shared with migraine and anxiety. Selective serotonin receptor inhibitors (SSRIs) might help in the treatment.

Cervicogenic Dizziness

There is a widely prevalent misconception that dizziness is cervicogenic and is related to cervical spine degeneration. Such a situation could arise only when there is significant altered proprioceptive input from the neck due to extensive facet arthropathy or cervical radiculopathy. The occurrence of compression of vertebral artery (VA) in the cervical spine is rare, and is not usually associated with the occurrence of isolated vertigo but manifests with other symptoms of brain stem involvement (neighborhood signs) as outlined earlier.

Drugs and Toxins

Aminoglycosides (streptomycin and gentamycin), diuretics, benzodiazepines, amiodarone, antipsychotics, zolpidem can cause dizziness.

Central causes of dizziness are causes related to the CNS and not the peripheral vestibular apparatus or the vestibular nerve. A normal neurological examination excludes a central process. 10% of the patients with involvement of the medial branch of posterior inferior cerebellar artery (PICA) may have isolated vertigo.

Head Impulse, Nystagmus and Test for Skew Examination

Head impulse test has been dealt with earlier.

Test for Skew

Cover test: Patient maintains gaze on the examiner's nose and the examiner alternatively covers each of the patient's eye. Positive result is indicated by deviation of one eye while it is being covered followed by correction on uncovering it **(Figs. 4A and B)**.

An array of central nervous system disorders can cause dizziness:
- Stroke
- Multiple sclerosis

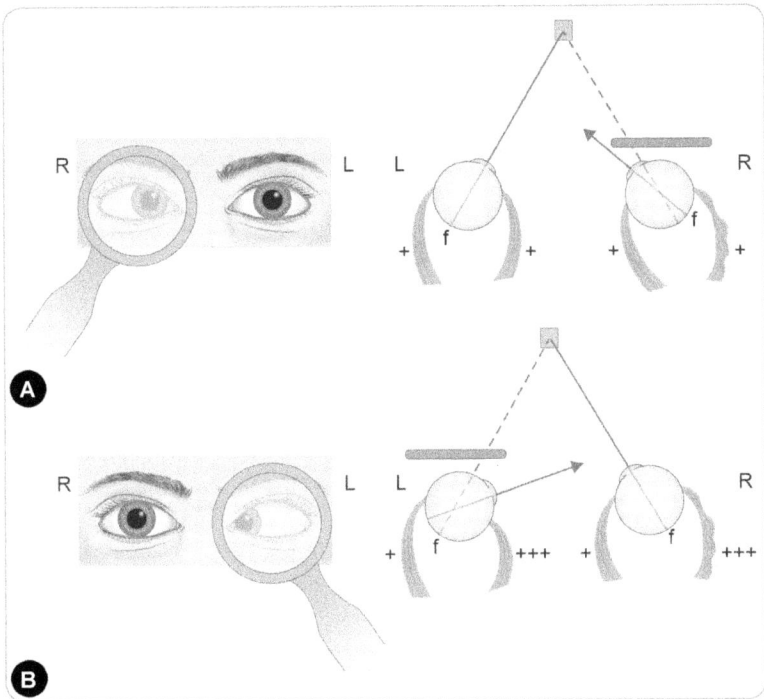

FIGS. 4A AND B: Right lateral rectus muscle palsy and primary and secondary deviation. (A) Left eye fixes on the object while the right eye is obscured by an occluder. It is shown that there is a minor right esotropia (primary deviation) (in this illustration, the opaque occluder is partially translucent, so that the reader can see where the covered eye is located, but the patient is unable to see through it). (B) The right paretic eye is fixated on the object while the left eye is covered. Despite having a weak right lateral rectus muscle, the right eye can focus on the object because the central nervous system overdrives that muscle. Due to the Hering law of dual innervation, the normal left medial rectus muscle is also overworked, which causes a significant secondary deviation or esotropia.
(f: fovea)

- Brain tumors
- Acoustic schwannomas
- Neurodegenerative disorders associated with dysautonomia
- Chiari malformations
- Head trauma (frequent cause)—postconcussion syndrome
- Migraine with associated dysautonomia

Central nervous system causes are to be considered, when dizziness is associated with other symptoms and neurologic signs, of motor, sensory, or cerebellar long tracts involvement or with other cranial nerves involvement. MRI is essential in this setting, to identify the cause and treat accordingly. Long-standing dizziness also needs imaging to exclude a structural abnormality.

CHAPTER 3

Seizures

INTRODUCTION

When a person turns up with a symptom suggestive of a seizure, the first objective should be to confirm whether the event was indeed a seizure, as there are several seizure mimics.

The diagnosis of a seizure is a clinical diagnosis that is made based on the description of the event. There is no test to establish that the event, was a seizure, apart from the history obtained from the patient, based on what the patient felt before and after the event, and also from an eyewitness as to what had happened during the event, as the patient would not remember what happened during the event except in the case of partial or focal seizures.

A video of the event, if it had been captured, or requesting the family members to take a video when such an event recurs, would help in establishing and confirming the diagnosis.

Video electroencephalography (EEG), i.e., recording the EEG at the same time as the patient is having a seizure which is also recorded on the video, is the only confirmatory investigation which would differentiate a seizure from a pseudoseizure and other seizure mimics. Video EEG synchronizes the electrical activity in the brain with the involuntary movements and helps to confirm a seizure. Generalized tonic-clonic seizure type is rather easy to diagnose based on the description given and needs to be differentiated from only pseudoseizures.

- Focal motor seizures (jerking of face, upper limbs, or lower limbs) are also easy to diagnose based on the description, though this may have to be differentiated from other involuntary movements such as myoclonus, dystonia, chorea, tics, and ballismus. Asking the patient to demonstrate the nature of the involuntary movement or taking a video of the movement would most often be helpful.
- It is the episode of isolated loss of consciousness (LOC), without involuntary movements or incontinence of bladder or bowel, and without tongue bite, which poses the maximal difficulty in diagnosis and so are the episodes associated with hyperventilation, when pseudoseizures would become the first diagnosis.

CONDITIONS WHICH COULD RESEMBLE A SEIZURE EPISODE

- *Loss of consciousness (LOC)* occurs not only with seizures but also with a number of seizure mimics, the common ones being:
  - Syncope
  - Transient ischemic attack (TIA)
  - Migraine
  - Falls in the elderly due to nonseizure events
  - Drop attacks
  - Psychogenic episodes
  - Movement disorders wherein falls occur, but the occurrence of associated LOC is not certain
  - Hyperglycemia and hypoglycemia
- *Sleep disorder*: Narcolepsy with cataplexy can be mistaken for a seizure. This is a condition with sudden collapse and rapid recovery to baseline mental status, with complete recollection of the event, and at times associated with emotional precipitants.
- *Syncope* is a sudden LOC due to reduced cerebral perfusion resulting in loss of postural tone with rapid return to baseline mental status; this could be due to cardiac, orthostatic, or neurocardiogenic causes.
  Precipitating factors of syncope are as follows:
  - Recent illness such as emesis or diarrhea, resulting in hypovolemia
  - Recent medication changes which could result in bradycardia, diuresis, and hypovolemia

- LOC following increase in vagal tone (coughing, defecation, micturition)
- LOC during physical exertion

Myoclonic jerking could occur in up to 90% of persons experiencing syncope.
- *Migraine*: Migraine with aura can be similar to focal seizures with visual symptoms or with generalized seizures prodrome. Complex migraine or migraine with basilar features can cause alteration in consciousness or LOC, mimicking a seizure. Sensory aura of migraine can mimic a sensory seizure.

Epileptic seizures which resemble one of the epilepsy mimics are called epilepsy chameleons (epilepsy in disguise).

Laboratory studies may be helpful at times in differentiating a seizure from nonseizure events if done immediately after the event. Serum prolactin is increased in 100% of tonic-clonic seizures and in about 84% of complex partial seizures, if serum is tested immediately after the seizure episode. The sensitivity of increased serum lactate is 88% and specificity is 87%. The specificity of increased serum creatine kinase is 85-100% and sensitivity is 15-88%. The serum levels should be measured within 10-20 minutes after a suspected event.

Seizures are of different types, and establishing the type of seizure will help in better management, as the efficacy of the chosen drug would vary with the type of seizures.

TYPES OF SEIZURES

Focal or partial seizures can be either simple or complex. Focal seizures are called simple when consciousness is not affected and can be motor, sensory, or autonomic. When altered sensorium is associated with partial seizures, it is referred to as complex partial seizures. The recent terminology is focal seizures with impaired awareness (FSIA).

Generalized seizures include the following:
- Absence seizures
- Myoclonic seizures
- Generalized tonic-clonic seizures
- Drop attacks

Seizures are broadly divided into:
- Focal or partial
- Generalized

} as mentioned above

The type of seizure has to be classified based on the description of the seizure event given by the patient or the eyewitness. Focal and focal seizures with impaired awareness might be a manifestation of an underlying structural abnormality, and hence imaging will be required to identify the cause of the seizures.

Generalized seizures can be further classified into:
- *Absence seizures* are characterized by an abrupt impairment of consciousness with no postictal deficit or confusion. The age of onset is between 5 and 15 years and the duration is brief, of <20 seconds. Hyperventilation will bring on these episodes and the EEG shows a characteristic 3 Hz spike and wave discharges of abrupt onset and termination, with no change in the background activity, and this is considered a pathognomonic feature.
- *Myoclonic seizures* are features of juvenile myoclonic epilepsy (JME) and progressive myoclonic epilepsy. JME has its onset in the 2nd and early 3rd decade of life, mostly between the ages of 12 and 18 years. The EEG shows a characteristic 3–6 Hz polyspike and wave changes, and an abnormality in chromosomes 6p and 15q has been identified to be associated with this condition.
- JME occurs generally early in the morning and is related to sleep deprivation, alcohol use, flashing lights, and social distress. A question would have to be asked specifically of the patient as to whether there are jerks of the arms and trunk, especially on getting up.

  Treatment, even without recurrence, is for an indefinite period, as it has the propensity to recur at any time and at any age. Valproic acid and levetiracetam are the drugs of choice and valproic acid is best avoided, if possible, in females in the reproductive age group. Clonazepam and zonisamide also control myoclonic jerks. Lamotrigine is also a first line drug especially in pregnancy with monitoring of blood levels.
- *Progressive myoclonic epilepsy* is a childhood-onset disorder characterized by recurrent myoclonic seizures and is usually associated with cognitive impairment. It indicates an underlying neurometabolic or genetic brain abnormality.
- *Generalized tonic-clonic seizures* can be primary, when it is a generalized seizure from onset, or secondary, when a focal seizure spreads in the brain to become generalized tonic-clonic seizures.
- *Primary generalized tonic-clonic seizures* are less common than secondary generalized seizures and could have a genetic

component as the etiological factor—genetic generalized epilepsies. Primary generalized seizures tend to occur in the early morning on arousal and occurs usually in the 2nd or early 3rd decade of life like JME.
- *Secondary generalized seizures* occur when the focal seizures and focal seizures with impaired awareness (FSIA) spread to adjacent areas, especially to the midline (thalamus), and become generalized.
- Focal seizures with impaired awareness are focal seizures, with alteration of conscious level, which may vary from impairment to total loss of cognition. The partial seizures, most of the time, comprise behavioral arrests or automatisms or auras, with loss of memory of the event, which could progress to total LOC and generalization.

  The auras may take the form of an epigastric sensation rising up, a feeling of abnormal sensation in the limbs, visual hallucinations, Déjà vu (familiarity with new places), or Jamais vu (unfamiliarity with known items or places). Experiential illusions could occur wherein the patient feels a strong sense of familiarity with scenes which she or he has never seen or experienced before and, on the contrary, a sense of strangeness about visual stimuli such as the face of a close relative or an experiential situation that should be familiar. These auras indicate the site of origin of the seizures, temporal, parietal, or occipital, depending on the nature of the stimulus.
- *Frontal lobe seizures* generally do not have an aura and are hypermotor and abrupt in onset. They are brief and occur as multiple episodes, which could be difficult to control.
- *Automatisms* consist of movement of the arms purposelessly, or lip smacking, chewing, and swallowing, which have to be specifically asked for from the eyewitness by demonstrating such movements.

MANAGEMENT

Patients with focal, partial, or focal seizures with impaired awareness (FSIA) seizures need to have imaging done to look for an underlying structural abnormality as stated earlier.

For those who have generalized seizures, namely absence, myoclonic, or generalized tonic-clonic seizures, occurring in the early hours and in association with certain electroclinical syndromes, an EEG is more informative as there are specific characteristics or signature features in the EEG to identify these specific types of seizures. EEG is, however, not a diagnostic test for seizures and could be normal in up to 50% of the patients.

Carbamazepine and oxcarbazepine are the drugs of choice for partial seizures, apart from lacosamide, a relatively new drug. Valproic acid would be the drug of choice for generalized seizures, be it absence, myoclonic, or primary generalized seizures. Ethosuximide is the drug of choice for absence seizures. Levetiracetam, lacosamide, and clobazam could be used for both partial and generalized seizures, mostly as add-ons. Difficult-to-control seizures may need to be worked up for surgical therapy. CENOBAMATE is a recent addition and most promising drug for focal seizures yet to be introduced in India.

DROP ATTACKS

Seizures are one of the causes of a drop attack, which is also termed atonic seizures or akinetic seizures. Usually, there is no LOC and the legs give way making the subject to fall or slump. Eyelids drooping and head dropping forward could be observed and jerky movements could sometimes occur. Refractory epileptic conditions such as Lennox–Gastaut syndrome and Dravet syndrome are common causes of drop attack seizures.

CHAPTER 4

Limb Weakness

INTRODUCTION

Muscle weakness can be due to either dysfunction of central nervous system or peripheral nervous system. Neurological examination helps in recognizing the pattern of weakness which is necessary for localization in the neuraxis.

WEAKNESS

Whenever a person presents with weakness of limbs, the following points will have to be asked for:
- Whether the weakness is in one limb, which is known as monoparesis,
- Whether it is unilateral, affecting both upper and lower limbs, which is termed hemiparesis, or
- Whether it is bilateral, affecting all four limbs, and is called quadriparesis

When only a part of the limb is involved, it is called focal weakness. Having detected a weakness, the next step is to find out whether this weakness has features of lower motor neuron (LMN) or upper motor neuron (UMN), even if it happens to be a focal limb weakness.

LOWER MOTOR NEURON

The features of an LMN lesion are:
- Decreased tone of the muscle
- Wasting of the muscle
- Fasciculation in the muscle
- Decreased or absent tendon reflexes

Of these, wasting and fasciculation would be present only when the lesion is chronic and hence in an acute lesion, the decision of whether the lesion is LMN or UMN would depend mainly on the tone and the state of the tendon reflexes. However, in a state of spinal shock associated with an UMN lesion, the tendon reflexes could be absent and the tone could be flaccid and hence it would be difficult to differentiate from a LMN lesion.

An increase in tone is easier to detect than decreased tone, and hence absence of increased tone and decreased or absent tendon reflexes would indicate a LMN involvement, while increased tone and brisk reflexes would indicate an UMN lesion.

Chronic LMN lesions may be associated with wasting and fasciculation. After establishing whether the weakness is due to LMN or UMN involvement, the next step would be to try to locate the site of lesion within the LMN or UMN.

The following would be the features of different sites of the lesion within the LMN:
- *Anterior horn cells*: The distinctive features of anterior horn cell involvement would be wasting and fasciculation with wasting being more in degree than the weakness and with differential involvement in the wasting and weakness of the muscles supplied by the same segment.
- *Roots:* Monoradiculopathy when the findings are in the distribution of a single root or polyradiculopathy when the changes are more diffuse, characterized by weakness, reduced tone, and reduced reflexes when acute, and with wasting in addition, if chronic in nature.
- *Plexus:* When the findings include sensory involvement and do not involve a specific myotome or a dermatome and are in the distribution of multiple motor and sensory nerves, a plexus involvement should be suspected. Reflexes are usually lost but at times can be retained in plexus lesions.
- *Nerves:* The weakness and wasting, if present, are in the distribution of the muscles innervated by the respective nerve or nerves. Tone and reflexes may or may not be affected and if

affected, they would be focal. Sensory involvement would be in the distribution of the nerve.
- *Neuromuscular junction (NMJ):* Fatigability, diurnal variation, and ocular and bulbar muscle weakness would be the key components of NMJ involvement with no wasting, fasciculation, or sensory involvement. The tone would be reduced in the affected muscles, and the reflexes are usually preserved in myasthenia gravis, while it is reduced or absent in Eaton-Lambert syndrome which is also a NMJ disorder.
- *Muscle:* Weakness will be the predominant feature without much of wasting. Reflexes would be diminished according to the degree of loss of muscle power. Muscle pathologies cause bilateral and symmetric manifestations with predominant involvement of proximal muscles.

MYOPATHIES

The most common pattern of muscle weakness in myopathies is symmetric weakness affecting predominantly the proximal muscles of the legs and arms, the so-called limb girdle (pelvic and pectoral girdles) distribution. The distal muscles can also be involved but usually to a lesser extent. The neck muscles can be affected as well as the ocular and bulbar muscles in both neuromuscular junction disorders (NMJDs) and muscle diseases. A knowledge of distribution of the muscle weakness and the disorders associated with such weakness would help in the diagnosis.

Disorders Causing Predominant Distal Muscles Weakness in Upper Extremities

- Inclusion body myositis (IBM)
- Myotonic dystrophy (MD)
- Welander's distal myopathy
- Scapuloperoneal syndrome including facioscapulohumeral dystrophy (FSHD)

In IBM, the wrist and finger flexors are involved early with relative preservation of the strength in wrist and finger extensors. In MD, weakness of the wrist and finger extensors occurs in contrast to the flexor weakness in IBM. Welander's distal myopathy is an autosomal dominant disorder occurring in the 5th decade of life and presenting as distal hand weakness, with weakness of thumb extensors spreading to the hand and later to involve the legs, resulting in thumb drop and foot drop. FSHD and scapuloperoneal syndrome have prominent winging of the scapula with peroneal muscle weakness and facial weakness.

Disorders Causing Predominant Distal Muscle Weakness in Lower Limbs

- *Autosomal dominant (AD)*:
  - Early onset—Laing myopathy
  - Late onset—Markesbery-Griggs myopathy
- *Autosomal recessive (AR)*:
  - Anterior compartment—tibial muscle—Nonaka, hereditary IBM
  - Posterior compartment—calf muscle—Miyoshi myopathy **(Figs. 1A and B)**

Other myopathies: IBM, MD, desminopathy, debranching enzyme deficiency.

Desminopathy can involve lower limbs, upper limbs, trunk and neck muscles, and facial and bulbar muscles and cause cardiomyopathy and respiratory muscle weakness. It is associated with mutation in desmin or Alpha B-crystallin.

Debranching enzyme deficiency in the adult form causes distal weakness affecting the calves and peroneal muscles with increased creatine phosphokinase (CPK).

Features which Help in the Diagnosis

Myopathies with Involvement of Scapular and Peroneal Muscles

- FSHD
- Scapuloperoneal dystrophy

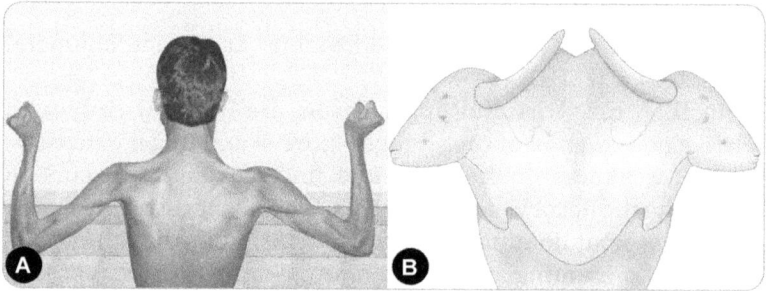

FIGS. 1A AND B: Calf heads on trophy sign in Miyoshi myopathy.

- Emery-Dreifuss myopathy
- Limb girdle— calpainopathy
- Pompe disease (acid maltase deficiency)

Myopathies with Ptosis and with or without Ophthalmoplegia
- MD—ptosis and facial weakness, no ophthalmoparesis
- FSHD—facial weakness, no ophthalmoparesis, ptosis in atypical phenotypes
- Oculopharyngeal muscular dystrophy (OPMD)—ptosis, ophthalmoplegia, dysphagia
- Chronic progressive external ophthalmoplegia (CPEO)—ptosis and ophthalmoplegia, no dysphagia
- Congenital myopathy (centronuclear myopathy)—ptosis and ophthalmoparesis

Myopathies with Bifacial Weakness
- MD
- FSHD
- Congenital myopathies of central core, nemaline

Myopathies with Dysphagia
- MD with reduced esophageal motility and esophageal dilatation
- OPMD
- Inflammatory myopathies
- Desminopathy

Myopathies Associated with Neck Muscle Weakness
- Inflammatory myopathies
- MD
- FSHD
- Pompe disease (acid maltase deficiency)
- Desminopathy

Myopathies Associated with Atrophy
Atrophy is more common in denervating neuropathies and anterior horn cell disease but can occur in muscle diseases as described under:
- Calpainopathies—generalized muscle atrophy
- Limb-girdle muscular dystrophy (LGMD)—preferential atrophy of hip adductors

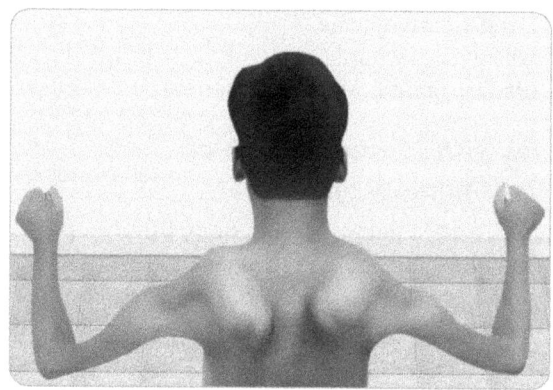

FIG. 2: Poly-Hill sign in facioscapulohumeral dystrophy (FSHD).

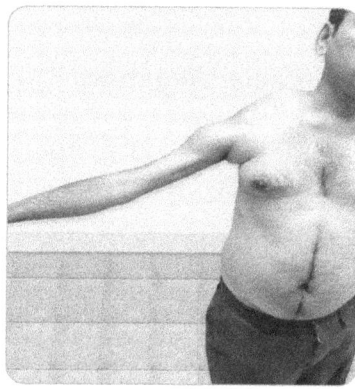

FIG. 3: Popeye arm seen in facioscapulohumeral dystrophy (FSHD).

- Calf and hamstring muscles atrophy in dysferlinopathy
- FSHD—wasting of the upper portion of deltoid, the arm muscle and the lower portion of deltoids and trapezius may be hypertrophic referred to as the "Poly-Hill" sign **(Figs. 2 and 3)**.
- MD—wasting of masseter, temporalis, and neck muscles gives rise to an elongated hollowed-out face (hatchet face) with a swan neck deformity.

Hypertrophy

True hypertrophy occurs in myotonia congenita and stiff person syndrome (SPS). Pseudohypertrophy of the calf muscles is seen in Duchenne muscular dystrophy (DMD), Becker's muscular dystrophy (BMD), and LGMD and also occurs in hypothyroid myopathy, amyloidosis, sarcoidosis, and neoplastic and inflammatory myopathy.

Myopathies Associated with Myalgias
- Osteomalacic myopathy
- Endocrine myopathies, especially hypothyroid
- Inflammatory myopathies
- Eosinophilia-myalgia syndrome
- Infectious myositis—viral, bacterial, fungal, parasitic
- Toxic myopathies due to medications and toxins

Myopathies according to age of onset:
- *At birth*: Hereditary myopathies, congenital muscular dystrophies, and congenital myopathies.
- *Presenting in childhood*: DMD, BMD, EDMD, dermatomyositis, infectious myopathies, and metabolic myopathies.
- *Presenting in adulthood*: Inflammatory myopathies, endocrine myopathies, FSHD, LGMD, and toxic myopathies.
- *In elderly*: IBM and OPMD.

The nature of weakness must be enquired as to whether the weakness is persistent or occurs episodically. Persistent weakness would indicate dystrophies and inflammatory myopathy, while episodic weakness is characteristic of periodic paralysis, metabolic myopathies, and NMJDs.

Features Related to Muscle Involvement

Cramps
Dehydration, hyponatremia, azotemia, hypothyroidism, adrenal insufficiency, renal and hepatic failure, and pregnancy are common causes of cramps.

Other causes include metabolic myopathies such as hypothyroid and McArdle's myopathy (myophosphorylase deficiency).

Cramps are uncommon in muscular dystrophy and inflammatory myopathies and are most common in motor neuron disease, bulbospinal form of spinal muscular atrophy (Kennedy syndrome) and chronic neuropathies, and radiculopathies.

Contractures
Contractures occur early in the course of the disease in Emery-Dreifuss muscular dystrophy (EDMD) and in collagenopathies such as Bethlem myopathy (keloids). They are late features in

DMD and in dermatomyositis. They differ from cramps in that the electromyography (EMG) shows no activity with contractures, whereas there are muscle discharges in cramps.

Myotonia

Myotonia refers to an impaired relaxation of muscle, exhibited most commonly in the eyelids and hand muscles, with difficulty in relaxing the handgrip or opening a bottle top and opening the eyelids after closing them tight. It can occur in hypothyroid myopathy and hyperkalemic periodic paralysis, apart from MD, congenital myotonia, and paramyotonia where it is the key feature.

The myotonia in myotonia congenita improves with exercise while in paramyotonia congenita, the myotonia worsens with exercise. In both these conditions, the myotonia worsens with exposure to cold temperatures.

Myoglobinuria

Myoglobinuria refers to the presence of myoglobin in urine which occurs with rhabdomyolysis or rapid destruction of the muscle. Myoglobin is released from the muscle which can cause renal failure when severe.

Acquired causes of myoglobinuria are as follows:
- Exposure to drugs and toxins such as alcohol, clofibrate, opiate, and statins.
- Heat stroke or prolonged fever, neuroleptic malignant syndrome (NMS), serotonin syndrome, snake venom poisoning, and trauma are the other causes.
- The familial causes include metabolic myopathies and malignant hyperthermia.

Myopathy Associations

Presence of:
- Keloid → Bethlem myopathy
- Lipomas → Mitochondrial myopathy
- Sensorineural hearing impairment → Mitochondrial myopathies, FSHD
- Optic atrophy or pigmentary retinopathy → Mitochondrial myopathy, FSHD
- Colorblindness → EDMD

- Cataracts → Myotonic dystrophy, MD, mitochondrial myopathy
- Coat's disease → FSHD

Motor system examination in myopathy can reveal wasting, hypertrophy, pseudohypertrophy, fasciculation, skeletal deformity such as pes cavus, and kyphoscoliosis, all of which can be picked up on inspection.

Most primary muscle diseases exhibit proximal, symmetric weakness of the muscles. Reflexes are retained till the late stages in myopathies except in mitochondrial disease wherein it could be lost early. Normally, the center of gravity of the body passes in front of the hip joint. Persons with back extensor weakness assume a lordotic posture, so that the center of gravity of the upper body passes behind the hip joints to stabilize the posture.

Creatine kinase (CK or CPK): Estimation of CK in serum is the most common and useful test performed for detecting patients with myopathic disorders. CK is elevated transiently in any disorder causing damage to the muscle such as trauma to the muscle, injections, contusion, viral infections, strenuous exercise, and seizures. It is elevated persistently in inflammatory and dystrophic myopathies. It may be normal or minimally elevated in mild or slowly progressive muscle diseases, end-stage myopathy, and endocrine and steroid myopathies. Statins, chloroquine, and cyclosporine ingestion can cause an increase in CK levels.

NEUROPATHIES

The neuropathy can be sensorimotor, motor, sensory, and/or autonomic, depending on the manifestation.

Symptoms indicating involvement of the autonomic nerves which escape our attention are:
- Erectile dysfunction
- Bowel and bladder involvement
- Postural hypotension
- Postprandial bloating
- Dryness of mouth
- Edema and coldness of extremities
- Sweating abnormalities

The following key aspects have to be determined when neuropathies are suspected, based on the history and examination.
- *Temporal profile of evolution*: Whether the neuropathy is acute, chronic, or relapsing and remitting

- *Which nerve fibers are involved*: Motor, sensory, autonomic, or a combination of these fibers
- *What is the distribution of the weakness*: Asymmetric or symmetric, focal or widespread, proximal or distal, or both

Large fiber sensory involvement causes tingling sensation, imbalance, areflexia, Romberg's sign, muscle weakness, impaired joint position sense (JPS), and vibration sense (VS). Small fiber sensory involvement results in burning pain, severe paresthesia, reduced pain and temperature sensations, retained reflexes, and normal JPS and VS.

Examination would reveal whether the neuropathy is sensory, sensorimotor, or motor; whether the distribution is distal, proximal, or both proximal and distal; and whether the autonomic fibers are also involved, which would help narrow down the differential diagnosis. Nerve conduction studies (NCS) could help identify whether the pathology is demyelinating or axonal which would further help in narrowing down the differential diagnosis.

The common causes of acute neuropathies when the duration is <4 weeks are:
- Acute inflammatory demyelinating polyneuropathy (AIDP) or Guillain-Barre syndrome (GBS) (predominantly motor)
- Mononeuritis multiplex (MNM) (sensorimotor)
- Paraneoplastic sensory neuropathy (sensory), which is less common
- Proximal diabetic neuropathy (motor) simulating chronic inflammatory demyelinating polyneuropathy (CIDP) but rather acute in evolution
- Porphyria (predominantly motor)
- Arsenic poisoning resulting in sensory neuropathy

Causes of Chronic Neuropathies

Diabetes mellitus, hereditary motor sensory neuropathy (HMSN), CIDP, multifocal motor neuropathy (MMN), toxic, infective, and nutritional and metabolic neuropathies are causes of chronic neuropathies.

The relapsing, remitting neuropathies are CIDP and hereditary neuropathy with susceptibility to pressure palsy (HNNP).

Some features on general examination which would be a clue to the etiology are:
- Anemia in vitamin B12 deficiency and clubbing in POEMS (Polyneuropathy, Organomegaly, Endocrinopathy, Monoclonal

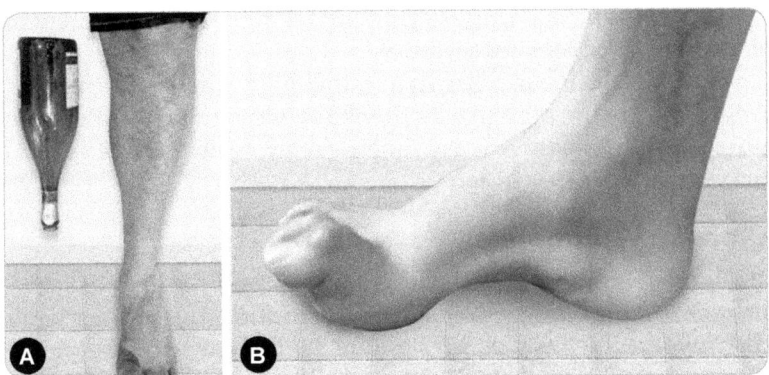

FIGS. 4A AND B: (A) Inverted champagne bottle appearance of leg; (B) hammer toes and high arched foot seen in hereditary motor sensory neuropathy (HMSN).

gammopathy, and Skin changes) and in paraneoplastic neuropathy
- Painless ulcer in leprosy, hereditary sensory neuropathy (HSN)
- High arched feet, hammer toes, claw hands, and inverted champagne bottle appearance of legs in HMSN **(Figs. 4A and B)**
- Hyperpigmentation of knuckles in B12 deficiency
- Skin lesions or skin changes noted in vasculitis, amyloid, and leprosy
- Mees line in the nails and raindrop pigmentation on the skin are seen with arsenic poisoning
- Burton's line on the gums occurring with lead exposure
- Curly hair in giant axonal dystrophy
- Loss of hair occurring with thallium toxicity
- Thickened nerves on palpation indicating leprosy, CIDP, and HMSN

The easily palpable nerves are the ulnar, greater auricular, common peroneal, and radial cutaneous nerves.

Common Neuropathies Encountered in Practice

Some of the common neuropathies encountered in practice are described below.

Leprous Neuropathy

Mononeuritis multiplex is the most common presentation of this treatable neuropathy and commonly affects the ulnar nerve, radial nerve, peroneal nerve, and branches of the facial nerve in the tuberculoid type and causes symmetrical nodular enlargement of the nerves in lepromatous leprosy.

Skin involvement with hypoesthetic or anesthetic patches would be a feature present with the above two varieties, while in the pure neuritic type there is asymmetrical involvement of peripheral nerves without a skin lesion.

Diabetic Neuropathies

The most common type of diabetic neuropathy is the distal sensory or sensorimotor polyneuropathy with stocking and glove type of distribution of sensory deficit signifying involvement of large nerve fibers according to their fiber length and termed as fiber length dependant neuropathy.

The other common presentation which is more troublesome for the patient is the painful sensory neuropathy, with burning sensation in the feet indicative of small fiber involvement.

Diabetic autonomic neuropathy (DAN) is more common than it is realized and causes erectile dysfunction, urinary symptoms, gastroparesis, and more importantly cardiac autonomic neuropathy (CAN).

Cranial nerves 7, 3, and 6 are the most common cranial nerves to be involved in diabetes in that order, causing cranial mononeuropathy.

Acute and Subacute Neuropathy of Guillain–Barre Syndrome or Acute Inflammatory Demyelinating Polyneuropathy

This condition is predominantly a motor neuropathy, usually affecting all four limbs causing muscle weakness involving the proximal muscles more than the distal. The weakness evolves subacutely over a period of usually a week to 10 days and is preceded by gastrointestinal or respiratory tract infections. Facial and bulbar muscles could also get affected.

Areflexia is a characteristic feature with or without mild sensory involvement. Cerebrospinal fluid (CSF) analysis is characterized by an increase in CSF protein with no increase in cells (albuminocytological dissociation). Demyelination on NCS is seen in typical presentations of GBS, but mixed axonal and demyelination changes and predominant axonal changes are also frequently encountered.

Chronic Inflammatory Demyelinating Polyneuropathy

Chronic inflammatory demyelinating polyneuropathy is a chronic neuropathy with more than 2 months of progressive or relapsing proximal and distal weakness with sensory involvement, areflexia, albuminocytological dissociation in CSF, and demyelination on NCS.

Inherited Neuropathies

Hereditary motor sensory neuropathy or Charcot-Marie-Tooth disease and hereditary sensory autonomic neuropathy (HSAN) are the common inherited neuropathies.

Toxic Neuropathies

Toxic neuropathies are due to drugs and heavy metals poisoning such as mercury, lead, thallium, and arsenic.

The differential diagnosis of this huge group can be narrowed down by ascertaining the type of neuropathy with the help of NCS, as most of the neuropathies are axonal except that due to diphtheria, chloroquine, and tacrolimus.

Distal symmetric, axonal, sensorimotor neuropathy: Most of the toxins or drugs cause such length-dependent neuropathy.
The drugs and toxins associated with the neuropathies are:
- *Motor-sensory neuropathy*: Amiodarone, tacrolimus, arsenic
- *Axonal motor neuropathy*: Organophosphates, lead, dapsone, vinca alkaloids
- *Sensory neuropathy*: Metronidazole, thalidomide, cisplatin, pyridoxine

LIMB WEAKNESS

Upper Motor Neuron

The features of a UMN lesion are:
- Increased tone in the muscles
- Brisk or exaggerated deep tendon reflexes (DTRs)
- Extensor plantar response
- Absent abdominal reflex
- Brisk jaw jerk if the lesion is bilateral and above the pons

There is no wasting or fasciculation in an upper motor neuron lesion unless it is associated with a LMN lesion also.

Once the weakness has been identified to be due to UMN involvement, its localization has to be established as the pyramidal tract involvement can be anywhere from the spinal cord to the cerebral cortex.

The level of the pyramidal tract involvement in the spinal cord is determined by the associated level of sensory involvement. If there is no sensory involvement, the level would have to be determined based on the DTRs.

A lesion will be localized in the thoracic cord if the reflexes are brisk or exaggerated only in the lower limbs and in the cervical cord or above it if the reflexes are brisk in both lower limbs and upper limbs.

A unilateral pyramidal lesion above or in the brainstem can be identified by facial nerve involvement and when it is bilateral by the presence of a brisk jaw jerk.

Brainstem lesions are usually associated with cranial nerve involvement apart from the involvement of pyramidal, sensory, and cerebellar tracts.

Lesions at the subcortical level between the midbrain and the cortex could be associated with extrapyramidal and visual field involvement. When the weakness is due to a cortical involvement, language and memory functions could also be affected. However, a pure cortical lesion does not usually cause weakness unless the lesion extends into the subcortical region.

Monoparesis

A LMN involvement causing a monoparesis is likely to be due to weakness of proximal muscles, or proximal and distal muscles, and is caused by a root or plexus involvement.

An UMN lesion can involve one limb due to a stroke, and this could involve an upper limb with UMN facial involvement, when it is called a faciobrachial paresis due to middle cerebral territory infarct. Lower limb involvement, a crural monoparesis, is less common and is due to anterior cerebral territory infarct.

In UMN lesions, distal weakness is more while in LMN lesions, proximal weakness would be more than or equal in severity to the distal weakness when the whole limb is weak.

CHAPTER 5

Speech Abnormalities

INTRODUCTION
Abnormalities in speech can be dysarthria or dysphasia or aphasia.

DISARTICULATION
Disarticulation refers to a disorder of articulation with no difficulty in comprehension or expression of words. Vowels, which are produced in the larynx, are minimally affected or not affected at all, and only consonants, which are produced by movements of lips, tongue, and pharynx, are mispronounced.

DYSARTHRIA
The different types of dysarthria are as follows:
- *Spastic dysarthria*, due to upper motor neuron (UMN) involvement of the bulbar muscles which results in a slurred speech with telescoping of words and is termed hot potato speech as it mimics the speech which would come out when there is hot stuff inside the mouth.
- *Ataxic speech or cerebellar speech*, due to cerebellar involvement resulting in the syllables being separated and is termed scanning or staccato speech. The words are broken with a pause between the syllables.

- *Monotonous or halting speech*, which occurs with extrapyramidal involvement as in Parkinson's disease where the speech is in a low tone without intonations.
- *Flaccid speech*, characterized with imprecise vocalization and a nasal voice, occurs with a lower motor neuron involvement of X and XII cranial nerves or when the bulbar muscles are affected in neuromuscular junction disorders or myopathies.

DYSPHASIA OR APHASIA

Dysphasia or aphasia refers to a defect of language, wherein the patient is not able to find or express words fluently or is not able to understand spoken words.

Nonfluent Dysphasia or Broca's Aphasia

In this type of aphasia, which is also termed expressive or anterior aphasia, comprehension is intact but spontaneous speech is broken and telegraphic with a few words and short sentences, leaving off adverbs and adjectives, though the meaning gets conveyed.

The lesion is in the inferior frontal gyrus due to involvement of the superior division of the middle cerebral artery (MCA).

Wernicke's Aphasia

In Wernicke's or receptive or posterior aphasia, comprehension is lost but spontaneous speech will be fluent and excessive with grammatical errors and meaningless words called neologism and is associated with paraphasias which is referred to as jargon speech. The lesion is in the superior temporal gyrus in the auditory association cortex and angular gyrus and is usually due to involvement of the inferior division of the MCA.

Global Aphasia

Global aphasia refers to the inability to comprehend as well as to express and is due to a large lesion involving Broca's and Wernicke's areas due to involvement of the internal carotid or proximal MCA.

Conduction Aphasia

In conduction aphasia, the person can speak and comprehend but cannot repeat what is told because the lesion involves the arcuate fasciculus which connects the Wernicke's (comprehension) area with the Broca's (expression) area and the information cannot pass from the comprehension area to the expression area and this occurs due to occlusion of the terminal branch of the MCA.

Note of caution: Before coming to the conclusion that a person is dysphasic, it has to be made certain that the person is conscious and not disoriented, or in delirium, as in these states the speech might appear to be dysphasic when actually the language areas are not involved.

Similarly, a person with Wernicke's aphasia could be misunderstood to be disoriented or psychic because the speech would be irrelevant and not understandable and also response inappropriate because of poor comprehension. Care should be taken in interpretation in the above situations.

Examination of an aphasic patient should include assessments of the following:
- Comprehension
- Fluency
- Repetition
- Reading
- Naming
- Writing

To test naming, objects are shown to the patient and he or she is asked to name them. The patient can have phonemic paraphasia wherein the subject is unable to pronounce the word properly or substitute it with wrong words, which is termed semantic paraphasia. The site of lesion with difficulty in naming is in the middle and inferior temporal gyri.

Reading is considered abnormal when the person has difficulty in comprehending the material given to be read, or when the fluency and pronunciation are affected. Difficulty in reading, known as alexia or dyslexia, occurs with lesions between the left occipital cortex and the posterior part of the corpus callosum when they are unable to read the given material.

Writing difficulty is called dysgraphia or agraphia and refers to the inability to write to dictation or copy printed material and may have mistakes in spelling, grammar, or the sequence of words. The lesion is in the middle frontal gyrus of the dominant hemisphere in patients with difficulty in writing.

CHAPTER 6

Visual Symptoms

INTRODUCTION

The common visual symptoms related to neurology are:
- Pain in the eye
- Blurring of vision
- Loss of vision

Pain in the eye can be an irritation or a burning sensation. Pain which is throbbing could be associated with a migraine headache when the internal carotid vessel is affected and the surrounding nerves are excited.

The pain could be aching or stabbing around the eye with neuralgias and with inflammatory lesions involving the orbit and periorbital regions. Other causes of pain in the eye include corneal abrasion, glaucoma, inflammatory lesion of the eye, trauma, and systemic and neurologic disorders.

Blurring of vision is complained of when the images are indistinct. The numerous causes could include a foreign body on the cornea, refractive error, medications, injury to the eye, and neurologic disorders.

Unilateral blurring occurs with ocular involvement, corneal abrasions, foreign bodies, cataract, and other lens changes. Other causes include central serous retinopathy, diabetic retinopathy, retinal vein occlusion, and neurological causes (optic neuropathies).

When a patient presents with loss of vision, the following details should be obtained:
- Is the visual loss unilateral or bilateral?
- Is it transient or persistent?
- Is it sudden or gradual?
- Is it painless or painful?

This information helps in formulating a differential diagnosis. The ocular causes of visual loss are:
- Retinopathies
- Vitreous abnormalities
- Macular involvement
- Cataracts

The neurologic causes of vision loss are:
- Inflammatory demyelinating optic neuritis (ON)
- Ischemic optic neuropathies
- Transient ischemic attack (TIA) involving the retina
- Tumors of the optic nerve and orbit

Apart from visual impairment, patients could also have visual field defects which are as follows:
- *Scotoma*, which is a small area of the visual field that is not seen. It can be central or cecocentral. Scotomas can be absolute or relative and can be positive or negative. In an absolute scotoma, the blind spot is totally blind and no light of any intensity is perceived within the scotoma. A positive scotoma is one where the person can perceive a patch blocking the vision. A central scotoma is one wherein the blind spot occurs in the center of the visual field looking like a black or gray spot for some, and for others it may be a blurred image.

  In a cecocentral scotoma, the visual field defect extends from the central vision to the natural blind spot. This field defect represents an insult to the cluster of retinal ganglion cells (RGC) called the papillomacular bundle. Scintillating scotomas are flashes of light or burst of lights commonly seen with migraine.
- *Hemianopias*: Loss or reduction in vision can be confined to one half or one quarter of the visual field and is called hemianopia or quadrantanopia. The type of field defects helps in the localization of the lesion.
  - Optic nerve lesions result in central scotoma or arcuate defect.

- Nerve lesions just anterior to the chiasma produce junctional scotoma due to ipsilateral optic nerve involvement along with the inferior contralateral crossing fibers.
- Chiasmal lesions produce a bitemporal hemianopia.
- Optic tract lesions produce incongruous hemianopic defects.
- Lesions of the optic radiation result in either quadrantanopia or hemianopia, mostly congruous defects, depending on the location and extent of the lesion, upper quadrant involvement with temporal lobe lesion, and lower quadrant involvement with parietal lobe lesion.
- Lesion of the striate cortex produces a homonymous hemianopia, sometimes with macular sparing, especially with vascular involvement.
- Superior or inferior cortical lesion causes inferior or superior altitudinal field defects, respectively.
- The causes of optic nerve involvement causing visual loss and/or field defects include:
    - Demyelinating diseases—multiple sclerosis (MS), neuromyelitis optica (NMO)
    - Nerve fiber layer damage as in hypertension
    - Toxins—methyl alcohol, quinine, ethambutol
    - Nutritional deficiencies
    - Vascular events
    - Glaucoma, which damages axon from the inferonasal and inferotemporal retina resulting in an arcuate defect known as arcuate scotoma

OPTIC NERVE LESIONS

Optic Neuritis

Optic neuritis causes loss or diminution of vision, most often in one eye associated with pain in the same eye. Assessment of the visual loss would include visual acuity, visual field, and examination of the optic fundi.

Pinhole test: The patient is asked to look through a pinhole and if the vision improves, the impairment is due to refractory errors and not due to nerve lesions.

Relative afferent pupillary defect (RAPD): The swinging flashlight test is done to look for the RAPD observed by swinging the flashlight from one eye to the other. The affected eye constricts less even though it senses the light when the light is thrown on the affected eye as pupils of both eyes constrict but not fully as there is a lesion in the afferent pathway. But when the light is thrown on the normal eye, both pupils constrict further as the afferent pathway is intact. As the flashlight is swung from eye-to-eye, the defective eye shows less constriction and the pupil dilates.

The visual acuity when tested with Snellen's chart is grossly diminished with desaturation of the red color. The fundus might be normal or the disc margin could be blurred, when there is papillitis. It is important to differentiate papillitis from papilledema as in both conditions, there may be edema of the discs but in papillitis there is associated gross loss of vision, while in papilledema vision is relatively spared.

Anterior Ischemic Optic Neuropathy

Anterior ischemic optic neuropathy (AION) could produce unilateral disc edema and gross visual loss. Ischemic optic neuropathy could be arteritic when there is inflammation of the artery supplying the optic nerve or nonarteritic when there is noninflammatory involvement of the artery supplying the nerve.

Other causes of unilateral disc edema could be optic nerve compression within the orbit and diabetic papillopathy.

Optic Atrophy

- Optic atrophy is another condition causing visual loss.
- The disc is pale with the margins clearly demarcated.

The common causes of optic atrophy include:
- Idiopathic optic neuropathies
- Demyelinating neuritis—NMO, MS
- Toxins—alcohol, tobacco, ethambutol
- Vitamin B12 deficiency
- Systemic lupus erythematosus (SLE)
- Optic nerve compression
- Leber's hereditary optic neuropathy (LHON)
- Mitochondrial disorder involving the retinal ganglion cells (RGC)

Papilledema

- It refers to the condition where there is swelling of the disc which is hyperemic with indistinct margins and with an absence of venous pulsation **(Fig. 1)**.

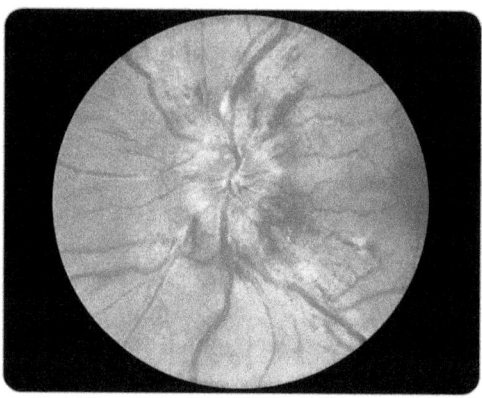

FIG. 1: Grade IV papilledema where there is obscuration of disc margin and swollen hyperemic disc.

- It is usually bilateral and indicates increased intracranial pressure.
- The visual acuity is usually normal, however, continuous unrelieved pressure on the optic nerve can lead to secondary atrophy of the disc with decreased vision.
- The visual field is affected minimally at the peripheries.
- Though papilledema is usually bilateral, unilateral disc edema can occur in one eye alone in the following conditions:
  ○ *Papillitis:* It is a term applied when the optic disc becomes edematous in one eye and is associated with dense loss of vision indicating inflammation of the optic nerve (optic neuritis).
  Causes of papillitis are as follows:
  – Demyelinating diseases such as MS, NMO, myelin oligodendrocyte glycoprotein (MOG) antigen-associated ON, or MOG-associated autoimmune disorders (MOGAAD) involving the optic nerves, brain, and spinal cord
  – Viral or other infectious diseases
  – Vascular causes as mentioned earlier
  – In many persons there is no apparent cause, and idiopathic optic neuropathy is considered
  – Papillitis is usually characterized by pain associated with movement of the eye, headache, and a rapid and progressive loss of vision.

1. *Foster-Kennedy syndrome* comprises ipsilateral optic atrophy due to compression of the optic nerve by the tumor per se (optic atrophy) and contralateral papilledema due to the raised intracranial pressure. Foster Kennedy syndrome is one of the important cause for progressive bilateral vision loss.
2. *Pseudo-Foster-Kennedy syndrome*: The findings are that one eye shows optic atrophy due to the old AION or ON and the other eye shows disc edema due to a fresh acute attack of AION or ON occurring sequentially as in NMO.

In both of the above conditions, one eye shows optic atrophy and the other eye disc edema. It is due to a tumor in Foster Kennedy syndrome on the other hand ON or ischemic optic neuropathy causes Pseudo Foster-Kennedy syndrome.

CHAPTER 7

Assessment of Higher Functions

INTRODUCTION

Assessment of higher functions begins with the most basic function, i.e., level of consciousness followed by basic cognitive domains like language, praxis and proceeds through complex functions like verbal reasoning, calculation, etc.

MENTAL FUNCTIONS

Cognition

Cognition refers to the total state of awareness and mental functioning ability of an individual. Cognitive assessment is essential to diagnose a cognitive disorder and once it is diagnosed, serial assessments need to be done to monitor the progression and to assess the response to treatment. The assessment should include the various domains of cognition that are affected and also the extent of involvement of each domain.

The domains of cognitive function assessed are:
- Attention and concentration
- Language
- Executive function
- Memory
- Praxis
- Gnosis

Aprosexia is the term given to describe the inability to focus and concentrate.

Attention is the ability to focus and concentrate on a stimulus. Some easy bedside tests to assess attention would be to ask the patient to:
- Spell "world" backward → dlrow
- Serially subtract 7 from 100, e.g., 93, 86, 79......
- Indicate by a tap whenever she/he hears a particular letter, by narrating a long series of letters
- Repeat initially a series of 6-7 numbers given to them and then to repeat the same numbers backward, i.e., from the last number given to the first number in that order, e.g.,

3, 7, 4, 9, 2, 5, 8 (forward)
8, 5, 2, 9, 4, 7, 3 (backward)

The structures associated with this test of attention are the reticular formation, thalamus, and the frontal cortex. The most common cause of decreased attention is diffuse brain dysfunction due to metabolic, toxic, or infective disorders. Multi-infarct state and brain injury with frontal lobe involvement are other causes of inattention and poor concentration.

Language

As we discussed earlier under language disorders, the examination of language function will include the assessment of:
- Naming
- Spontaneous speech
- Comprehension
- Repetition
- Reading and writing

Spontaneous Speech

Spontaneous speech or verbal fluency assessment is done by asking the person to speak at his or her normal speed. Normal word output is 200 words per minute. When word output is <50 per minute it is considered nonfluent. If the word output is fast >200 per minute, the condition is called logorrhea.

Comprehension

Comprehension is tested by:
- Asking the patient to close the eyes or put out the tongue and see whether he does it.

- Asking the names of various parts of the body or objects which is made further complex, by asking the subject to point to 3 or 4 objects in sequence as mentioned.
- Asking the subject to answer yes or no to simple and complex questions, e.g.,
  - Could ask the person to answer yes or no to the place where he/she is at that time by asking whether he/she is in a:
    - House
    - Theater
    - Hospital
    - Hotel

    And wait for a Yes or No answer to each clue.
  - Can ask whether carrot is a fruit? And ask him or her to answer Yes or No.
  - Can ask the person to answer Yes or No to what part of the day it is at that time by giving clues—morning, afternoon, evening or night.

  These also are tests of attention and orientation.

Repetition

Repetition is tested, by asking the patient to first repeat a word and then a sentence, and finally one of the popular repeat phrases is given and the subject is asked to repeat it, e.g., no ifs and/or buts, or an equivalent phrase coined in the vernacular.

Naming

Objects are shown and their colors are asked to be named, and the difficulty and errors are noted.

Reading and Writing

These are tested independently with words and sentences.

Memory

Principally the following types of memories are tested:
- *Immediate memory*: This is also a test of the attention and depends on the integrity of dorsolateral frontal cortex.

  The patient is given a five digit number or telephone number and is asked to repeat it. Alternatively, the person can also be given the names of three or four unrelated words including an

abstract one, and asked for the words to be repeated, e.g., wind, boy, box, and size.
- *Recent or short-term memory* can be tested by asking the subject to recall the numbers and the words given earlier, after 5 minutes.

The patient can be asked the details about the two previous meals he or she has had, and who were the visitors to his or her house the previous day. A short story might be narrated at the start of the examination and the subject asked about some aspects of it, at the end of the rest of the examination.

Recent memory or short-term memory is a function of the medial temporal lobe, namely the hippocampus and it is the earliest memory defect noted in Alzheimer's disease.
- *Remote or long-term memory* is of two types: Explicit or declarative and implicit or nondeclarative.

Explicit memory can be episodic or semantic. To test episodic explicit memory, the patient is asked details about his personal life of the past, namely his/her school teacher's name, school's name, date of birth, and the date of marriage. Episodic memory is not affected in Alzheimer's disease, and it is represented in the neocortex.

Semantic explicit memory involves testing the general knowledge that is knowledge about leaders, the political scenario, color, and the differences among animals. Semantic memory is a function of the anterior and inferior temporal lobe and is involved in the semantic form of frontotemporal dementia.

Procedural memory is the implicit type or nondeclarative memory related to learned or acquired skills, consisting of knowledge of previous experience, e.g., driving a bike, playing cricket or football, or doing a pole vault. Procedural memory is impaired in late degenerative Parkinson's disorders, as basal ganglia and the cerebellum are dysfunctional and can also happen with traumatic brain injury (TBI) to these areas.

LOBAR FUNCTIONS

Lobar functions can be divided into assessment of the following lobes:
- Frontal
- Temporal
- Parietal
- Occipital

Frontal lobar functions assessment can be split into assessment of the following areas of the frontal lobe:
- Motor area
- Premotor area
- Frontal eye fields
- Dorsolateral prefrontal cortex (DLPFC)
- Orbitofrontal cortex (OFC)
- Supplementary motor area
- Anterior cingulate gyrus

The motor area or primary motor cortex is the precentral gyrus or Brodmann area 4 **(Figs. 1A and B)**. This is tested by asking the patient to grip the examiner's fingers (hand grip test). Weakness of

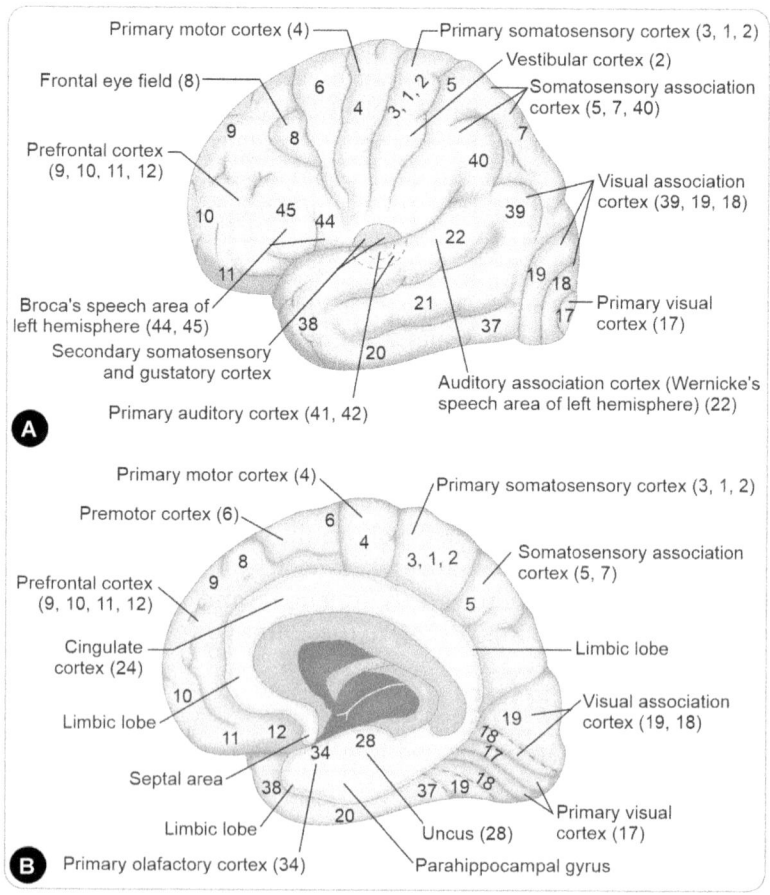

FIGS. 1A AND B: Brodmann areas.

hand grip indicates involvement of this motor cortex or subcortical areas therein.

Premotor cortex is Brodmann area 6, and is the area anterior to the motor cortex which is involved with sensory motor integration. Cortical or subcortical lesions in this area result in apraxia (limb kinetic) and difficulty in performance of movements smoothly.

This is tested by asking the patient to touch the other fingers of his or her hand with the thumb, in rapid succession. The speed and ease of doing this is assessed. A simple and easy test for apraxia is to ask the patient to rotate a coin between the thumb and other fingers. A normal individual will be able to do >12 rotations in 1 minute. A limb kinetic apraxia is identified if only <10 rotations are possible.

Frontal eye fields are situated in Brodmann area 8. The function of this area is to direct the patient's gaze to the opposite side. If this area is damaged, the patient's gaze is directed to the same side.

Dorsolateral Prefrontal Cortex

This is the largest part of the frontal lobe and includes Brodmann areas 9, 10, and 46 and is responsible for the executive functions, attention, and working memory.

Planning an action by integrating all sensory inputs and selecting the most appropriate response and performing it sequentially is the function of this area.

Tests of Dorsolateral Prefrontal Cortex

1. **Executive function:** To test this function, the following may be done:
   - The patient is asked to narrate the days of the week and months of the year backward.
   - The subject is asked how he would plan a trip to a mentioned place and what arrangements he would do for the same to undertake the trip.
   - The patient is asked to carry out a complex command, like picking up a piece of paper from the table and folding it into two or four and put it on the table again.
2. **Verbal fluency test (VFT):** Category of fluency is tested by asking the patient to give names of animals, fruits, vegetables, and also a list of words starting with a particular letter such as A, S, and B, etc., within 1 minute.

Dementing illness and traumatic brain injury are the principal causes of impairment on this test and the word list generated is <16.

3. **Attention tests:** Attention is tested with the following tasks:
   - *GO-NO-GO test*: Ask the patient to hold up one finger if the examiner holds up two and two fingers if the examiner holds up one. Test out first to ensure his or her understanding of the task and after ensuring that perform 10 trials.

   A failure to respond correctly and just repeating (echopraxia) suggests a lack of normal response inhibition. Inhibitory control is mediated by orbitomedial aspects of the frontal lobe (areas 11, 12).

   The rules are then changed to ask the patient to show the index finger when the examiner shows two fingers and do nothing when the examiner shows one finger. The second test is the actual GO-NO-GO test.
   - *Antisaccade task*: After ensuring eye movement and the visual fields are intact, the patient is asked to move his or her eyes contralateral to the stimulus, which could be wiggling a finger. If the left hand wiggles, the patient's eyes should move approximately an equal distance to the right.

   Failure to do this task reflects dysfunction in the DLPFC or a lesion interrupting the pathway between this frontal region and the superior colliculus.

4. **Cognitive set shifting:**
   Trail making test (TMT): This is used as a diagnostic tool for assessing cognitive shifts. It contains two parts **(Figs. 2 and 3)**.
   Part A: Patient connects 25 numbered circles sequentially.
   Part B: Numbers 1–13 and letters A–M must be connected in alternating progression from 1-A, 2-B to M-13.
   Total score is the time in seconds spent to complete each part.

   Trail making test tests the cognitive flexibility which is a function of the dorsolateral and medial prefrontal cortex (which was mentioned earlier).

5. **Letter fluency test:**
   Word generation—Thurstone test: The patient is asked to generate as many words as possible in 1 minute starting with a given letter and the words should not consist of proper names or adjectives or adverbs and the patient should be able to generate at least 8 words in a minute.

   This is also known as letter fluency test of frontal lobe function lateralizing to the left frontal lobe.

CHAPTER 7: Assessment of Higher Functions

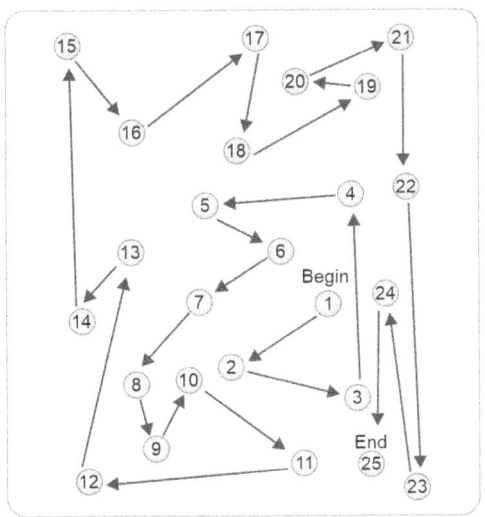

FIG. 2: TRAIL A test.

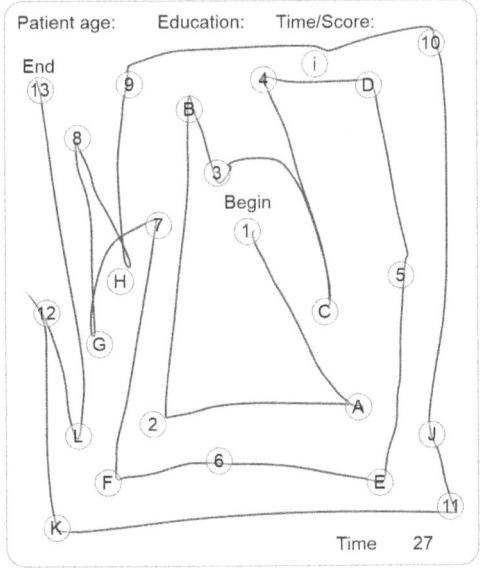

FIG. 3: TRAIL B test.

Semantic category fluency test: Listing out the names of animals or fruits or vegetables (category specific)—the semantic category fluency tasks test the temporal lobe function rather than frontal (mentioned earlier under VFT).

6. **Other tests:**
   - *Attention and concentration test*: All cognitive test performances depend on the status of the patient's attention and concentration. The tests for assessing attention and concentration have been dealt with earlier and hence are not repeated here.
   - *Fist-Edge-Palm test*: This test was described by Luria as a three-step motor program test of frontal lobe function. The patient is first asked to make a fist with his hand, then placing the edge of the hand and later laying the palm of the hand on the table.

     The test is considered abnormal if the patient is unable to do the movements sequentially.
   - *The applause test*: This is a test of perseveration. The patient is instructed to clap his hands three times after being demonstrated.

     It is considered abnormal if the patient continues to clap more than four times and it is a specific indicator of progressive supranuclear palsy or Parkinsonism states with frontal lobe involvement.

Orbitofrontal Cortex

The assessment of orbitofrontal cortex is done by observation of the patient's appearance and behavior, and by noting whether it conforms to the accepted social customs or whether there is lack of concern for the same like making silly or indiscreet jokes at inappropriate situations. Inhibitory control is mediated by this area.

Anterior Cingulate Cortex

This is Brodmann area 24 and is concerned with motivation in an individual. Patients with lesions involving the anterior cingulate area are apathetic and also mute and need assistance to feed themselves. Usually seen with multi-infarct state and psychiatric disorders.

Frontal Release Reflexes

The grasp, sucking, and palmomental reflexes which occur in babies and later get inhibited with the development of the frontal lobes, surface again with damage occurring to the frontal lobes either due to trauma or disease. The frontal release signs assume greater significance when they occur in young people and when they are unilateral.

PARIETAL LOBE FUNCTIONS

Praxis

The ability to perform skilled movements is called praxis and the inability to do so in spite of normal cognition and normal motor and sensory functions is called apraxia.

The engram for skilled limb movement resides in the left inferior parietal lobule for most right-handed persons. These engrams get converted to motor programs in the premotor cortices. Hence, left frontal lobe lesions near the supplementary motor and premotor cortices can cause limb apraxia (area 6 of Brodmann) apart from a lesion involving the left inferior parietal lobule.

Patients who have frontal lobe lesions can be apraxic for skilled limb movement without losing the movement or having the knowledge of it. This can happen with involvement of supplementary motor area, and convexity lesions, in addition to parietal lesions.

Praxis can be tested by asking the patient to pantomime the use of real tools such as a comb, toothbrush, screwdriver, or do a specific motor act such as coughing or blowing out a match. This is termed ideomotor apraxia.

Buccofacial apraxia occurs when patients cannot perform movements with the mouth or lips and they have separate localization, separately close to the Broca's area.

Callosal apraxia occurs with anterior cerebral artery strokes with unilateral left thumb apraxia and difficulty in performing simple tasks such as buttoning, cooking, and typing all previously learned movements.

Ideational apraxia refers to the inability to perform a goal-directed sequence of movements, with no difficulty in executing the individual components of the sequence, e.g., asking the patient to pick up a pen which has a cap and to write using it, and observe how the person starts writing with that pen. The perception of the object's purpose is lost.

The patient is asked to write a letter on a sheet of paper and then fold and put it in an envelope, write the address, seal it for posting, and affix a stamp similar to the one done for examination of the DLPFC functioning assessment. Sequencing-related problems are usually seen when the person is confused or demented.

Constructional apraxia refers to the inability to copy or draw an image correctly. The ability to successfully copy a line drawing, which involves seeing the diagram, processing the same visually (gnosis), and executing using motor function (praxis), is a test for gnosis and praxis.

Patients with damage to the left hemisphere tend to preserve the contents but oversimplify, by drawing figures and omitting details when drawing from memory. Systematically arranging the parts of their drawing will be difficult for them.

Right hemisphere involvement causes asymmetric or distorted drawings with hemispatial neglect, and omission of objects on one side of the picture namely, the left side.

Dressing apraxia: The patient would have difficulty in wearing his clothes and buttoning properly, which is caused by lesions of the parietal lobe.

Gerstmann's Syndrome

Gerstmann's syndrome consists of a combination of difficulties such as:
- Doing simple calculation (acalculia)
- Impaired writing (dysgraphia)
- Impaired finger naming (finger anomia)
- Left–right disorientation with difficulty in identifying the side
- Acalculia, dysgraphia, finger anomia, and right–left disorientation is associated with damage to left inferior parietal lobule

Hemispatial neglect occurs with right parietal lobe lesion (nondominant hemisphere).

Right hemisphere is concerned with directing attention to the entire extrapersonal space whereas the left hemisphere directs attention mostly within the right hemispatial space. Hence, unilateral left hemisphere lesion does not give rise to contralateral neglect since the right hemispherical attentional mechanism can compensate for the loss. Unilateral right hemisphere lesion gives rise to severe contralateral hemispatial neglect because the unaffected left hemisphere cannot compensate.

Patients with right parietal lobe lesion may fail to shave, groom, or dress on the left side and can neglect to eat what is on the left side of the plate and also fail to read the left half of a sentence.

BEDSIDE TESTS FOR PARIETAL LOBE

Clock Drawing Test

All the numbers are crowded on the right side with the left half being blank inside the circle **(Fig. 4)**.

Line Bisection Test

This is another test of parietal lobe function. A line is drawn and the subject is asked to bisect it. Line is not bisected equally with the left half being neglected and right half alone being bisected **(Fig. 5)**.

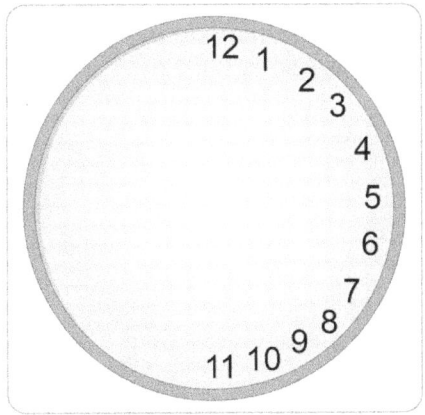

FIG. 4: Clock drawing abnormality—all numbers crowded on right side.

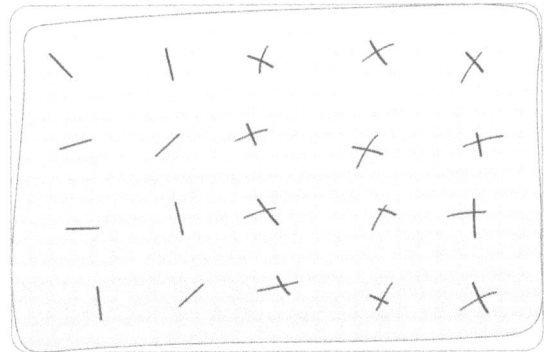

FIG. 5: Line bisection test—right half alone being bisected and left side neglected.

Balint's Syndrome

Features of Balint's Syndrome

SOAP—Simultagnosia, Optic ataxia, oculomotor Apraxia, Parietal lobe lesion is a useful mnemonic to remember the clinical features.

In simultagnosia, complex scenes are not grasped entirely and the focus is only on a small part of the imagery (missing the forest for the tree). Missing to reach out to an object or target accurately is called optic ataxia, while oculomotor apraxia refers to an inability to visually scan the environment orderly.

Balint's syndrome **(Fig. 6)** occurs with bilateral dorsal parietal involvement as it happens with bilateral watershed infarctions between the middle and posterior cerebral artery territories. Superior sagittal sinus thrombosis, hypoglycemia, and atypical forms of Alzheimer's disease can also give rise to Balint's syndrome.

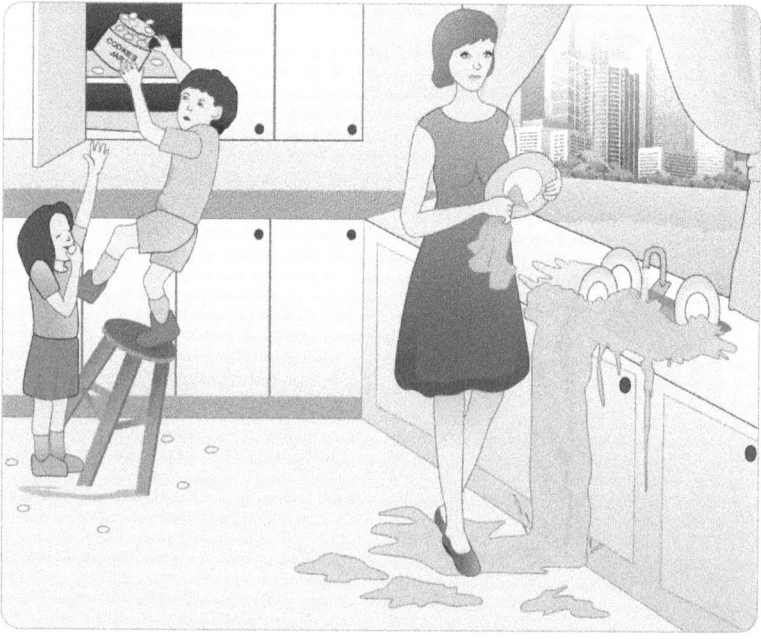

FIG. 6: The cookie theft picture where patients suffering from Balint's syndrome fail to see all but one of the simultaneously presented objects at the same location.

OCCIPITAL LOBE FUNCTIONS

Visual agnosia refers to the difficulty or impairment of identification of known objects, e.g., keys, rings, bangles, window, and collar.

Agnosia has to be differentiated from nominal aphasia, wherein also the patient may not be able to give the name of an object; if the patient is able to describe the object or demonstrate its use, then it is unlikely to be agnosia as visual perception is present and it suggests a nominal aphasia.

Prosopagnosia refers to the inability to identify faces of well-known celebrities, by looking at their photographs.

Color agnosia refers to not being able to identify and differentiate various colors. These defects occur with involvement of the visual association cortices areas 18 and 19 of Brodmann.

CHAPTER 8

Assessment of Sensorium

INTRODUCTION

The first step before assessing the higher functions is to evaluate the level of consciousness of the patient, which can be considered as the following states:
- Alert, when the person is in a fully awake state with normal response to external and internal stimuli.
- Drowsy, when the patient is not fully alert and drops off to sleep even while being examined.
- Stuporous, when the patient responds to only persistent or intense painful stimuli.
- Comatose, when the patient is unresponsive to any kind of stimuli.

The reticular activating system (RAS) extending from the brain stem to the cortex, through the thalamus, is concerned with maintaining normal sensorium. Consciousness requires an interaction between the RAS of the brainstem and the cerebral cortex. The RAS is responsible for arousal or alertness, and the cerebral cortex relates to consciousness of self and the environment.

It should be known that the individual's awareness of self is judged by the person's responses to external stimuli, both motor and verbal. While awareness refers to the qualitative aspects of functioning mediated by the cortex and includes cognitive skills such as attention, sensory perception, explicit memory, language, task execution, and temporal and spatial orientation, wakefulness describes the quantitative level of consciousness.

A comatose state can be defined clinically as a state with an inability to consistently follow a one-step command and can also be defined as a state with a score of <8 on the Glasgow Coma Scale (GCS) lasting for >6 hours with varying severity.
The clinical features of a person in a comatose state are:
- Inability to voluntarily open the eyes
- Scores between 3 and 8 on the GCS
- Irregular breathing
- Lack of response to physical (painful) or verbal stimuli
- Depressed brainstem reflexes such as pupils poorly reacting to light, or impaired vestibulo-ocular reflexes (VOR) or oculocephalic reflex (OCR)
- A nonexistent sleep wake cycle

GLASGOW COMA SCALE

Teasdale and Jennett developed a system to assess the level of consciousness in patients with head injury which is widely applied to score patients in coma due to any cause.

The GCS is scored in relation to eye, motor, and verbal response (EMV).
The scores are given as follows:
- *Eye response (E)*:
  - 4-spontaneous eye opening
  - 3-opening eyes to verbal command
  - 2-opening eyes to pain stimulus
  - 1-not opening the eyes to any stimulus

Maximum score for eye response (E) = 4
- *Motor response (M)*:
  - 6-obeys commands
  - 5-localizing pain stimulus and warding it off
  - 4-withdrawal response to pain
  - 3-flexor response to pain
  - 2-extensor response to pain
  - 1-no motor response to pain

Maximum score (M) = 6
- *Verbal response (V)*:
  - 5-oriented
  - 4-confused
  - 3-inappropriate words
  - 2-incomprehensible words
  - 1-no verbal response

Maximum score (V) = 5
Total score E + M + V = 4 + 6 + 5 = 15
If the score is <8, intubation is required. Though the GCS is the most widely used scoring, in assessment of coma, it has limitations especially in intubated patients as the verbal response cannot be assessed and hence an alternative has been devised.

FOUR

The acronym of FOUR is Full Outline of UnResponsiveness (Four score).

It is a clinical grading scale designed for assessment of patients with impaired level of consciousness developed by the neurocritical care team at the Mayo Clinic.

Four score is a 17-point scale ranging from 0 to 16. A decreasing score indicates worsening of the level of consciousness as it is with the GCS.

The four domains assessed are:
1. Eye response
2. Motor response
3. Brainstem reflexes
4. Breathing pattern

The need for developing this scoring system was the difficulty with assessing verbal response in intubated patients and hence GCS may not be able to give an accurate assessment of the conscious level.

Eye Response

- 4—eyelids open and eyes tracking or blinking
- 3—eyelids open but eyes not tracking
- 2—eyelids closed but open to a loud noise
- 1—eyelids closed but open to a painful stimulus
- 0—eyelids remain closed even on giving a painful stimulus

Motor Response

- 4—can show thumbs up, fist or peace sign on request
- 3—localizing response to pain
- 2—flexion response to pain
- 1—extension posturing response to pain
- 0—no response to pain, or presence of generalized myoclonus and status epilepticus.

Brainstem Reflexes
- 4—pupil and corneal reflexes are present
- 3—one pupil is wide and fixed
- 2—pupil or corneal reflexes are absent
- 1—pupil and corneal reflexes are absent
- 0—absent pupil, corneal, and cough reflex

Respiration or Breathing Pattern
- 4—not intubated, regular breathing pattern
- 3—not intubated, Cheyne-Stokes breathing pattern
- 2—not intubated, irregular breathing pattern
- 1—intubated and breathes above set ventilator rate
- 0—breathes at set ventilator rate or apnea

Conditions which affect the content of consciousness such as aphasia or major cognitive impairment (dementia) are likely to be confused with states of altered level of consciousness.

Acute confusional state (ACS) due to altered level of consciousness has to be differentiated from dementia due to altered content and this can be done by evaluating the following features are given in **Table 1**.

LOCKED IN SYNDROME

Due to quadriplegia and pseudobulbar palsy brought on by the disruption of corticospinal and bulbar pathways, the patient is awake, has sleep waking cycles, and meaningful behavior in the form of eye movements, but this is isolated in this state (de-efferented state). The only remaining movements are those of the eye or eyelids, but in cases with total locked in syndrome, these

TABLE 1: Features of acute confusional state (ACS).

Features	ACS	Dementia
Level of consciousness	Impaired	Not impaired
Course	Acute to subacute and fluctuating	Chronic, steadily progressive
Presence of autonomic hyperactivity	Often present	Absent
Prognosis	Usually, reversible	Usually, irreversible

Coma-like syndrome and related states; or disorders of consciousness (DOC).

movements may be paralyzed. The EEG is usually normal in this state, which is brought on by ventral pontine involvement.

Minimally Conscious State

The prognosis is better in this state than it would be for someone in a persistent vegetative state (PVS) if the patient has intermittent periods of wakefulness and awareness but is not able to communicate phrases. However, they might be able to follow simple instructions and speak a few meaningful words.

Persistent Vegetative State

In this state, the patient lacks awareness and is not able to communicate or has purposeful behavior. The sleep wake cycle is, however, preserved but there is no intellectual activity or social interaction. In both cerebral hemispheres, the white and gray matters are extensively damaged yet the brainstem is still intact.

After a traumatic brain injury (TBI), this state is known as a PVS if it lasts for >4 weeks. If it lasts for nearly a year, it is known as a permanent vegetative state, in which the metabolism falls between 40 and 50% of its normal level and the prognosis is worse.

CHRONIC COMA

Chronic coma is typically caused by localized brainstem lesions or cortical or white matter damage following neuronal or axonal injury. The patient is not aware of himself or their surroundings, and does not open eyes to stimuli. Gray matter metabolism falls between 50 and 70% of the typical range.

BRAIN DEATH

It is the irreversible cessation of all activity and functions including the involuntary activity necessary for life. Different countries have different standards for brain death, but the clinical evaluations are always the same and include:
- Loss of all brainstem reflexes; and
- Evidence of ongoing apnea in a patient who is permanently comatose.

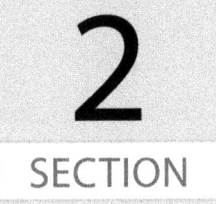

SECTION 2

Overview of Common Neurologic Disorders

CHAPTER 9: **Stroke**

CHAPTER 10: **Autoimmune Neurologic Disorders**

CHAPTER 11: **Movement Disorders**

CHAPTER 12: **Infections of the Nervous System**

CHAPTER 13: **Dementia**

CHAPTER 9

Stroke

INTRODUCTION

Stroke is a leading cause of mortality and more importantly, morbidity.

Stroke can be ischemic or hemorrhagic. Stroke should be suspected when a person presents with an acute or sudden onset of neurologic deficit, characterized by weakness of limbs and lower part of face, most often on one side. This might be associated with speech difficulty which could be a dysphasia or a dysarthria or a visual disturbance which is usually a visual field deficit. Other associated features are dizziness, headache, and altered sensorium depending on the site and size of the lesion.

ISCHEMIC STROKES

Ischemic strokes can be cardioembolic, or thromboembolic due to atherosclerotic occlusion.

Embolic strokes are secondary to cardiac or artery to artery embolism.

Cardioembolic strokes are more common in the anterior circulation territory. Some characteristic features of an embolic stroke are:
- Sudden onset with peak deficit at onset which might remain or clear quickly due to dissemination of the embolus
- Seizure occurrence at onset

- Dysphasia being the predominant or exclusive deficit
- Subpial site of infarct on imaging

Thrombotic occlusion occurs in the small vessel and large vessel and is the most common form of stroke.

The more common large-vessel strokes involve the middle cerebral and internal carotid arteries or posterior cerebral and posterior inferior cerebellar artery [large vessel occlusion (LVO) or large artery occlusion (LAO)] in the anterior and posterior circulation respectively.

Hemiparesis and language disturbance with upper motor neuron (UMN) facial paresis of varying degree of severity of involvement are the key features of middle cerebral artery strokes.

Differential involvements of upper limb, lower limb, and face with language involvement are features of cortical stroke, while more equal involvement of upper limb and lower limb without language involvement is indicative of subcortical stroke **(Figs. 1A to C)**.

Unilateral visual loss associated with abovementioned deficits on the contralateral side indicates internal carotid artery occlusion on the side of the visual loss.

Crossed hemiparesis, i.e., ipsilateral cranial nerve involvement with contralateral limb weakness or cerebellar signs and bilateral involvement with or without alteration of sensorium, suggests a posterior circulation stroke involving the brain stem.

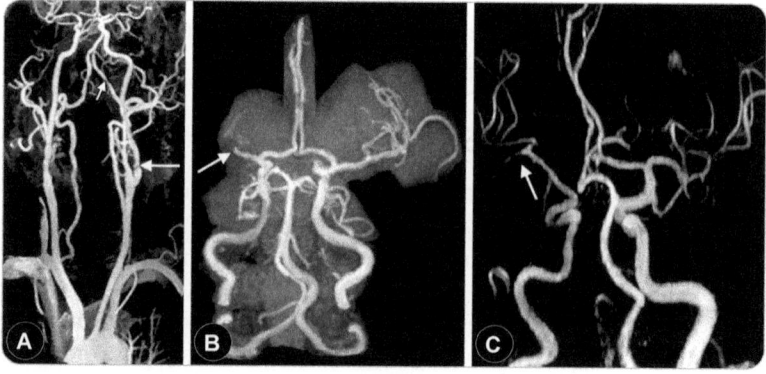

FIGS. 1A TO C: (A) Magnetic resonance angiography (MRA) of the carotid and vertebrobasilar circulations shows stenoses in proximal left internal carotid artery (large arrow) and distal left vertebral artery (small arrow); (B) MRA showing a complete occlusion (arrow) of the proximal M1 segment of the right middle cerebral artery (MCA); (C) right MCA distal occlusion (arrow).

DIAGNOSIS

Neurologic deficit, which is acute in onset, and is not progressing beyond a few hours, and is remaining static or improving, is either a stroke or a demyelination. The age of onset, the setting, and to some extent the clinical features would help in differentiating the two, but the confirmatory test is magnetic resonance imaging (MRI) of the brain. It should be noted that computed tomography (CT) scan may be negative in 40% and MRI in up to 20% of strokes termed as CT scan and MRI negative strokes, respectively in the hyperacute phase.

The diagnostic investigation of choice would be the MRI with MR diffusion and apparent diffusion coefficient (ADC) images, and should be looked for diffusion–FLAIR (fluid-attenuated inversion recovery) mismatch. However in stroke, the quickest and useful investigation would be CT angiogram (CTA) and every center which has a CT scan should have the software for a CTA so that the patient need not have to be shifted to a MR center for MRI and magnetic resonance angiography (MRA). CTA itself would give the necessary information on the size of infarct and the site of the vessel involvement and also the extent of collaterals to plan further management.

Computed tomography scans are more widely available and it just needs only an added software to have the angiogram done in the same sitting which at most would take 10 more minutes but it would save a lot of time in transporting the patient to a center with MR facility and bringing him back or take to another hospital for further treatment, all of which would be a waste of precious time.

As all of us know that time saved is brain saved, leading to the adage "Time is Brain" and the definite treatment should be given within 3 hours with tenecteplase (TNK) or within 4½ hours with alteplase [tissue plasminogen activator (tPA)]. That treatment with TNK has to be given within 3 hours is under scrutiny and it has now become an accepted practice to give TNK up to 4½ hours like alteplase, and this would soon be incorporated into the guidelines.

If thrombolysis is ineffective, and if there is a LVO, then mechanical thrombectomy needs to be done in centers which have the facilities for doing the same. To know whether it is a large vessel involvement or not, an angiogram is required, either CTA or MRA to check the site of blood vessel involvement.

It is in this context that the hospital having a CT scan should also have the facility for CTA so that the patient need not have to be shifted to a MRI facility thereby saving time for the start of treatment. A person with a large vessel occlusion should be shifted to a center where mechanical thrombectomy can be done [comprehensive stroke center-(CSC)].

Thrombolysis is the most effective current treatment recommended and will have to be carried out within the stipulated time. It has been established now that TNK is better suited for our country than alteplase because of the lesser cost and ease of administration, and also because of the equal, if not better response. TNK is now manufactured in India.

TENECTEPLASE

Tenecteplase is a genetically modified variant of alteplase with greater fibrin specificity and a longer half-life that permits bolus administration. Single intravenous (IV) bolus injection over 10 seconds with a dedicated IV line is given with no other medications being concurrently injected or infused. TNK caused better reperfusion in the trials conducted.

Trials with TNK are:
- *EXTEND 1A trial*: IV TNK 0.25 mg/kg (maximum dose 25 mg bolus); this is a lower dose trial instead of the initially recommended 0.4 mg/kg.
- *EXTEND 1A TNK part 2*: The dose of 0.4 mg/kg dose of TNK does not confer an advantage over the 0.25 mg/g dose. There are several ongoing clinical trials on TNK vis-à-vis alteplase and the results are awaited. These are TASTE, ATTEST-2, TEMPO-2, and TWIST trials.

Tenecteplase is manufactured in India and marketed as TENECTASE and the dose is 0.2–0.25 mg/kg and should be given IV within 3 hours of onset of stroke as a bolus injection which is being extended to within 4½ hours now.

Alteplase, the other thrombolytic agent, is costlier but can be given up to 4.5 hours IV at a dose of 0.9 mg/kg. 10% of the dose is given as bolus and the rest 90% given as infusion over 1 hour with monitoring in intensive care unit (ICU).

As mentioned earlier, the vascular occlusion can be in a large vessel or a small vessel. LVOs do not respond well to thrombolysis and at present, we have the option of doing mechanical thrombectomy for these patients to minimize the deficits. For the best results, thrombectomy should be done early, in <8 hours though the time limit can be extended up to 24 hours. The facilities for such treatment are expanding and is available in almost every city now.

It is for this reason that a CTA or MRA needs to be done as early as possible to determine the site of occlusion, and to assess the status of collateral supply. If the occlusion is in a large vessel, i.e., in the internal carotid or the first or second division of the middle cerebral artery, then mechanical thrombectomy would be the best option of treatment and should be planned to be done within 8-12 hours.

Under these circumstances, it would be best to thrombolyse with TENECTASE bolus and mobilize patient to a center where mechanical thrombectomy can be done following the GIVE and GO principle instead of the DRIP and SHIP policy where in alteplase is given over 1 hour as infusion and then the patient is shifted to the center where thrombectomy is available. Treatment with tenectase which is given as a bolus over 10 seconds saves >1 hour of valuable time compared to alteplase.

The pial (leptomeningeal) collateral circulation is a key determinant of functional outcome of mechanical thrombectomy after a large-vessel ischemic stroke. Patients with good collateral blood flow have benefit even up to 24 hours after stroke onset, whereas those with poor collateral flow show evidence of less or no benefit.

The concept of "collaterome" represents the elaborate neurovascular architecture within the brain that regulates and determines the compensatory ability response, and the outcome of cerebrovascular pathophysiology. The concept involves the entire cerebral circulatory system including arteries, veins and microvessels and incorporates interaction between the cerebral vascular architecture, cerebral blood flow (CBF) dynamics, tissue metabolism, and neuronal function. Cerebrovascular reserve plays a key role in the outcome.

"BE FAST" is the mnemonic for stroke detection and emergent treatment:
    B—Balance, dizziness
    E—Visual impairment
    F—Face
    A—Arm
    S—Speech
    T—Time

ASPECTS SCORE ON COMPUTED TOMOGRAPHY SCAN

Alberta Stroke Program Early CT Score (ASPECTS) is a 10-point quantitative score used to assess early ischemic changes on noncontrast CT scan. It provides a reliable and reproducible assessment of early ischemic changes in persons suspected to have acute LVO in the anterior circulation.

Calculation of the ASPECTS score: Each area of gray-white loss constitutes 1 point for deduction.
Subganglionic nuclei (below the basal ganglia level):
 M1—frontal operculum—1
 M2—anterior temporal lobe—1
 M3—posterior temporal lobe—1
Supraganglionic nuclei (above the basal ganglia):
 M4—anterior MCA—1
 M5—lateral MCA—1
 M6—posterior MCA—1
Basal ganglia (at basal ganglia level):
 Caudate (c)—1
 Lentiform (l)—1
 Insular (i)—1
 Internal capsule (IC) posterior limb—1
 Total ASPECTS score—10

A score of 7 and above indicates a good prognosis with thrombolysis, i.e., if more than three regions are involved, the prognosis is not good **(Figs. 2A and B)**.

HEMORRHAGIC STROKES

Unlike ischemic strokes which are confined to arterial territories, hemorrhagic strokes can extend in any direction and do not respect borders.

Intracerebral hemorrhage (ICH) and subarachnoid hemorrhage (SAH) are the two types of hemorrhagic strokes.

Subarachnoid Hemorrhage

Subarachnoid hemorrhage should be suspected in a person with sudden severe headache, known as "thunder clap" headache, with pain extending to the neck and going down the back. The presence of associated vomiting and meningeal signs indicates the diagnosis, which can be confirmed by a CT scan of the brain.

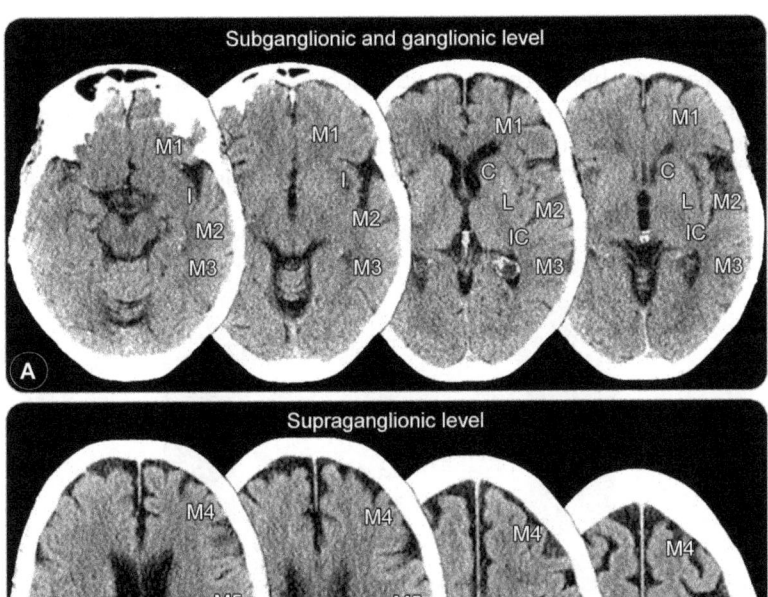

FIGS. 2A AND B: ASPECTS (Alberta Stroke Program Early CT Score) score illustrations.

This is a neurological emergency needing ICU care, and four-vessel angiogram should be done as early as possible before the patient rebleeds and deteriorates to find out the presence of an aneurysm and the site of the bleed. If there is an aneurysm, it has to be managed early before it rebleeds and hence the urgency in management.

Seizures can occur with SAH and the other dreaded complication is vasospasm resulting in shutting off of the blood supply in large vessels causing neurologic deficits. Obstruction to CSF pathway results in hydrocephalus and increase in the intracranial pressure, which would need surgical intervention.

Syndrome of inappropriate antidiuretic hormone secretion (SIADH) or cerebral salt wasting (CSW) causing hyponatremia would have to be anticipated and managed **(Fig. 3)**.

Intracerebral Hemorrhage

Intracerebral hemorrhage usually occurs due to hypertension, or rupture of an aneurysm or arteriovenous malformation (AVM) or a cavernoma (vascular anomalies). In the elderly, parenchymal hemorrhage (lobar) can occur due to amyloid angiopathy **(Figs. 4A to F)**.

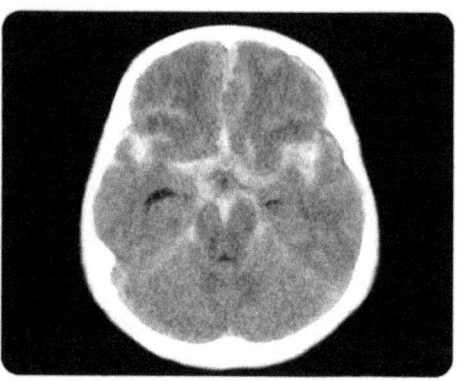

FIG. 3: Subarachnoid hemorrhage in the basal cisterns.

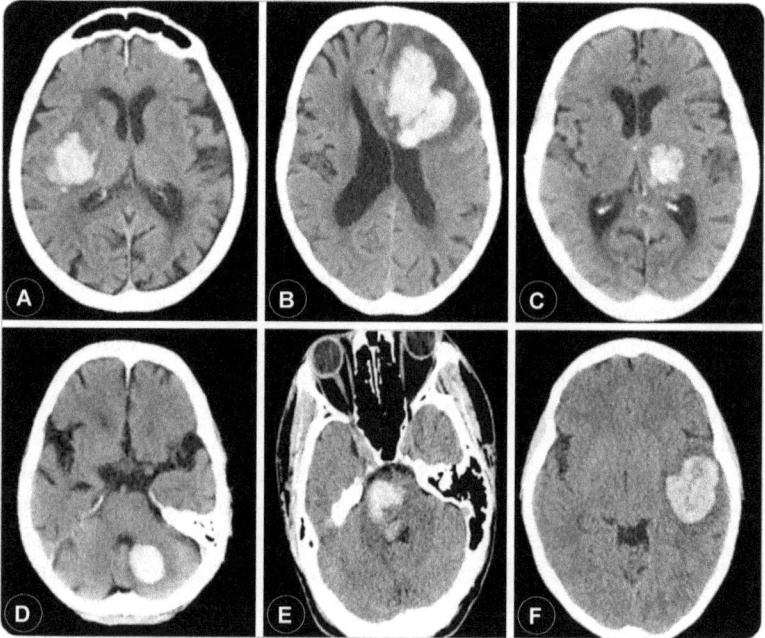

FIGS. 4A TO F: Intracranial hemorrhage in (A) right basal ganglia, (B) left frontal lobe, (C) left thalamus, (D) left cerebellum, (E) pons, and (F) left temporal lobe.

Cerebral hemorrhage is a medical neurologic condition, treated medically by physicians and the role for surgical intervention is limited to doing the following procedures in the given situations:
- Third ventriculostomy, when there is blood in the third and fourth ventricles causing hydrocephalus
- Evacuation of the clot (hematoma) when it is superficial, and close to the cortex, if the patient shows progressive deterioration
- Decompressive craniectomy, which would be required with large hemorrhages associated with gross mass effect
- Apart from the above three scenarios, surgical intervention is seldom required.

Medical management would be:
- Regulation of blood pressure
- Management of increased intracranial pressure when present, with osmotic and loop diuretics
- Observation of the course of the deficit for appropriate intervention when required

TRANSIENT ISCHEMIC ATTACKS

Transient ischemic attacks (TIAs) are focal neurological deficits occurring transiently and clearing spontaneously. Most often these deficits last for <1 hour, though by definition, the term includes deficits up to 24 hours. TIA is a warning event and may signal the onset of a full blown stroke later.

Up to 15% of persons could have a stroke within 3 months after a TIA and in 50% of these, strokes occur within the first 2 days. TIA is a medical emergency.

Diffusion-weighted MRI should be done to exclude an infarct as up to one-third of clinical TIAs could have an infarct on diffusion MRI, and >30% of these could progress to a stroke in 3 days. Hence, if an infarct is seen on diffusion MRI, it is better to thrombolyse, provided the patient is within the time window for thrombolysis.

Persons with a TIA should be evaluated with duplex studies of carotid and vertebral arteries, and if there is evidence of critical stenosis in these vessels, they should be evaluated further with angiographic studies for planning endovascular therapy (EVT).

Medical management would be with antiplatelet agents and statin, apart from the treatment of the risk factors.

The capsular warning syndrome is a term used to describe recurrent stereotyped lacunar TIAs. This syndrome is associated with a high risk of developing a completed stroke. The presumed mechanism for this syndrome is angiopathy of a lenticulostriate artery. Antiplatelets, heparin, pressors, and thromobolytics have all been used to treat patients with capsular warning syndrome.

CEREBRAL VENOUS SINUS THROMBOSIS

Cerebral venous sinus thrombosis (CVST) can present as seizures, thunderclap headache, hemiparesis, hemianopia, and dysphasia.

Sagittal and lateral sinus thromboses manifest with features of intracranial tension (ICT), namely headache, vomiting, papilledema, and deficits such as paraparesis and hemiparesis, with or without unilateral or bilateral sensory symptoms **(Figs. 5A to D)**.

Cavernous sinus thrombosis manifests with cranial nerves involvement and with chemosis and proptosis. Posterior cavernous sinus thrombosis or inferior petrosal sinus thrombosis may cause palsies of 6th, 9th, 10th, and 11th cranial nerves. Superior petrosal sinus causes 5th nerve palsy. Superficial thrombosis of cortical veins causes large superficial hemorrhagic infarction. Thrombosis of Vein of Labbé produces infarction of the superior temporal lobe and thrombosis of Vein of Trolard results in infarction of the parietal cortex. Cortical surface veins take "cork-screw" appearance in venous phase of the angiogram in venous thrombosis.

Deep Cerebral Venous Thrombosis

Occlusion of the vein of Galen and of the internal cerebral veins cause bilateral thalamic infarcts resulting in inattention, spatial neglect, akinetic mutism, and apathy. MRI shows a large bicircular region of signal change that encompasses the thalami with reversible edema and venous congestion **(Figs. 6A to D)**.

Treatment of Cerebral Venous Sinus Thrombosis

Anticoagulation with heparin and oral anticoagulants (OACs)—vitamin K antagonists or direct nonvitamin K antagonist OAC. Low molecular weight heparin (LMWH) followed by oral AC, warfarin or direct thrombin inhibitors.

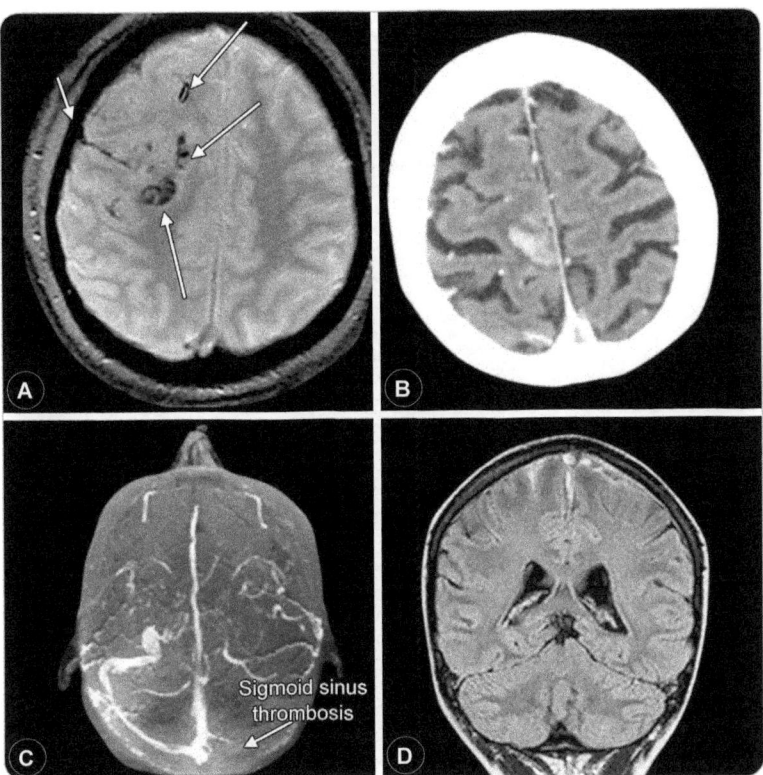

FIGS. 5A TO D: (A) Large arrows showing blooming in T2-weighted gradient resonance sequence magnetic resonance imaging (MRI) suggestive of cortical vein thrombosis; (B) empty delta sign on contrast computed tomography (CT) suggestive of superior sagittal sinus thrombosis; (C) small arrow showing absence of filling of left sigmoid sinus in MR venogram suggestive of sigmoid sinus thrombosis; (D) absence of flow void in superior sagittal sinus in FLAIR (fluid-attenuated inversion recovery)—MRI which suggests superior sagittal sinus thrombosis.

Nonvitamin K antagonists are termed variously as:
- NOAC—Novel oral anticoagulant
- TSOAC—Target specific oral anticoagulant
- DOAC—Direct oral anticoagulant

Warfarin is a vitamin K antagonist and inhibits vitamin K epoxide reductase factors 7, 9, 10, 11.

The nonvitamin K antagonist is dabigatran which directly inhibits factor 2A thrombin inhibitor.

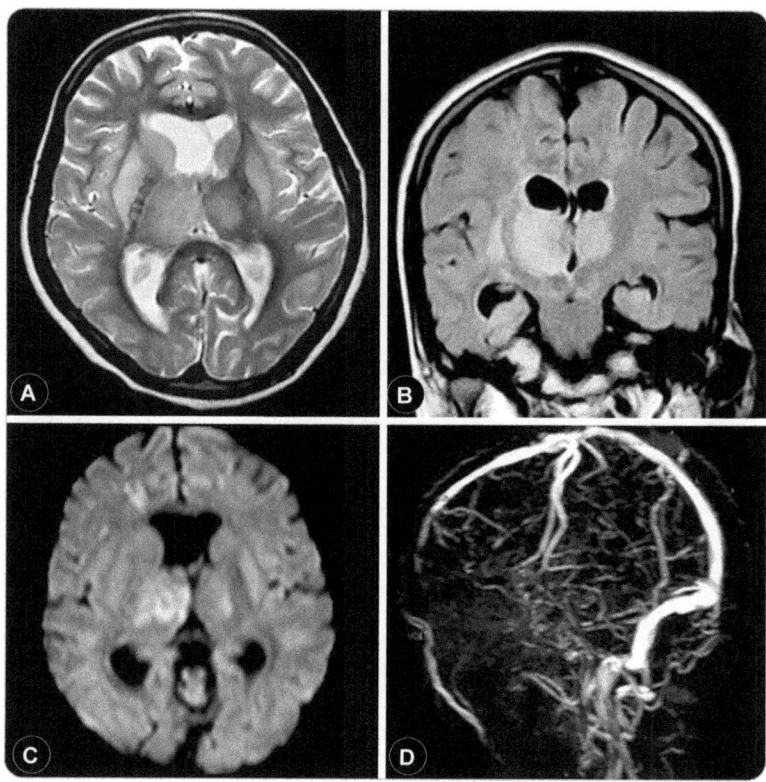

FIGS. 6A TO D: T2 axial (A) and FLAIR (fluid-attenuated inversion recovery) coronal (B) brain magnetic resonance imaging (MRI) showing hyperintensity in bilateral thalamus and basal ganglia with diffusion restriction (C). MR venography (MRV) reveals nonvisualization of deeper venous system suggestive of deep cerebral venous thrombosis (CVT) (D).

Rivaroxaban, apixaban, and edoxaban directly inhibit factor 10 A.

Why are NOACs so Appealing?

Bleeding is not more with NOAC though it is difficult to reverse, if it occurs. Bleeding occurs more with mechanical valves **(Table 1)**. Unlike warfarin and Acitrom it does not need monitoring of INR.

Bridging with Low Molecular Weight Heparin

This is generally not necessary due to the quick onset and offset of NOAC, and is required only in patients with high thrombotic

TABLE 1: Features of warfarin and novel oral anticoagulants (NOACs).

Warfarin	NOACs
High maintenance	More predictable
Impacted by dietary vitamin K	Not impacted by dietary vitamin K
Narrow therapeutic index	More constant pharmacokinetics
More drug interactions	Fewer drug interaction
Delayed pharmacodynamic onset	Quick onset of action <12 hours

risk, and in patients on warfarin who are planned for doing minor procedures. Interruption may not be needed for any anticoagulation use.

The following drugs are to be avoided with NOAC except for edoxaban (which is not much used) ketoconazole, fluconazole, heparin, ticagrelor, and rifampin.

Exercise caution in giving these drugs:
- Clopidogrel and other antiplatelet agents, verapamil, and diltiazem
- *Dose of NOACs*:
  ○ Dabigatran—150 mg bd
  ○ Edoxaban—60 mg od (not in use)
  ○ Apixaban—10 mg bd for 1 week followed by 5 mg bd
  ○ Rivaroxaban—20 mg od

CHAPTER 10

Autoimmune Neurologic Disorders

INTRODUCTION

Recent recognition of antibody-mediated nervous system disorders has led to research into antibody-mediated psychiatric illness such as schizophrenia and autism as well. The autoimmune neurological disorders can be categorized into the following groups.

AUTOIMMUNE VASCULITIS

Primary angiitis of the central nervous system (PACNS) is an inflammatory disease of brain affecting the cerebral blood vessels leading to a wide range of signs and symptoms including focal neurologic deficits, cognitive impairment, and psychiatric manifestations. If diagnosed and treated early, the inflammation could be reversible.

The differential diagnosis is distinctly different for angiography positive and angionegative PACNS subtypes, and differs depending on the age, there are 2 groups—(1) childhood PACNS and (2) adult PACNS.

Disease subtypes have been identified, each with a unique clinical course, neuroimaging results, and histological characteristics. Novel and conventional biomarkers including von Willebrand factor antigen and cytokine levels can be utilized to diagnose and characterize the subtype and disease activity.

The subtypes and activity of the disease should be taken into account when treating PACNS. In addition to immunosuppression, it would also contain medications to treat the symptoms and aid in recovery.

AUTOIMMUNE MOVEMENT DISORDERS

This covers a broad range of neurological conditions that can manifest alone or in conjunction with more widespread autoimmune encephalitic illness.

A wide spectrum of movements can occur ataxia, hypokinesia, and hyperkinesia such as myoclonus, tics, chorea, and other dyskinesias. The autoantibody targets are also diverse and include neuronal surface proteins such as synaptic proteins namely N-methyl-D-aspartate (NMDA), γ-aminobutyric acid (GABA), α-amino-3-hydroxy-5-methyl-4-isoxazolepropionic acid (AMPA), leucine-rich glioma-inactivated 1 (LGI1) and glycine receptors, and antibodies to intracellular proteins or antigens. These antibodies to the intracellular antigens are markers of a CNS process mediated by CD 8+ cytotoxic T cells.

The following disorders namely (1) Stiff-person syndrome (SPS) and (2) progressive encephalomyelitis with rigidity and myoclonus (PERM) are autoimmune movement disorders always.

When antibodies are found in serum and cerebrospinal fluid (CSF), such as when Purkinje cell cytoplasmic antibody (PCA-1) autoimmunity is present, this should prompt a search for malignancy as a possible cause. There are, however, some antibodies, such as glutamic acid decarboxylase-65 (GAD65) antibodies, where a paraneoplastic etiology is extremely unlikely and immunotherapy may help the patient recover **(Figs. 1A to D)**.

AUTOIMMUNE SLEEP DISORDERS

Sleep disorders are linked to a range of autoantibodies, some of which are paraneoplastic.

Intense insomnia and rapid eye movement sleep behavior disorder (RBD) can be caused by Morvan syndrome and limbic encephalitis associated with voltage-gated potassium channel complex antibodies, particularly against *Caspr2* and *LGI1*, respectively.

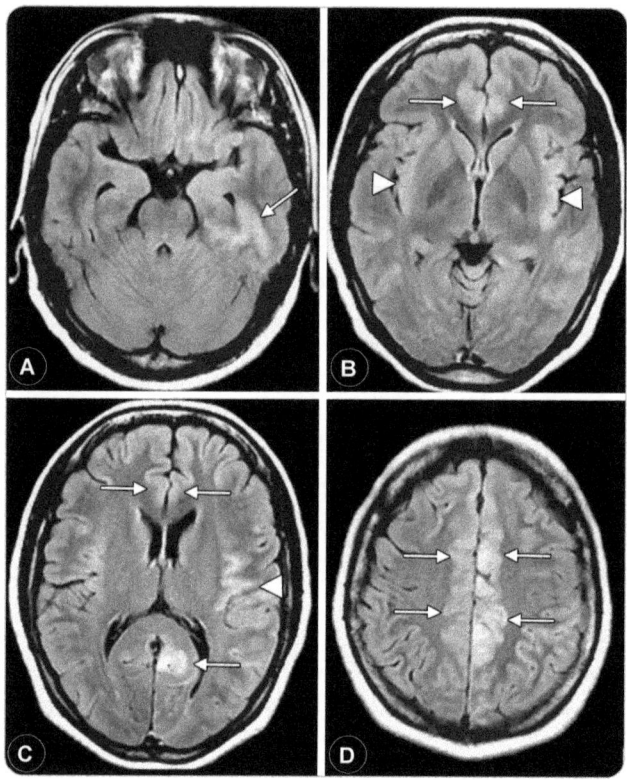

FIGS. 1A TO D: Magnetic resonance imaging (MRI) demonstrating T2-FLAIR hyperintensity in the left inferior temporal lobe (A), left > right insular cortex (B and C), and left > right cingulate gyrus (B to D) in anti-NMDAR encephalitis patient.
[FLAIR: fluid-attenuated inversion recovery; NMDAR: anti-N-methyl-D-aspartate (NMDA) receptor]

Narcolepsy can occur in conjunction with other signs of hypothalamic dysfunction in people with neuromyelitis optica (NMO) and aquaporin-4 (AQP4) antibodies, sometimes even as the first symptom.

Anti-NMDA receptor antibody encephalitis is linked to central sleep apnea and central neurogenic hypoventilation.

Stridor, hypoventilation, and obstructive sleep apnea are the main symptoms of a tauopathy linked to *IgLON5* antibodies.

The hypothalamus may be affected by paraneoplastic diseases, which can lead to sleep disorders, most notably narcolepsy and REM sleep behavior disorder in people who have *Ma1* and *Ma2* antibodies. Patients who have antineuronal nuclear antibody type 2 (ANNA-2) (Ri) might develop stridor.

Recent onset narcolepsy has high titers of antistreptococcal or other antibodies, suggesting that narcolepsy may have an autoimmune basis.

AUTOIMMUNE MYELOPATHIES

A diverse collection of immune-mediated spinal cord diseases with a wide range of differential diagnoses are known as autoimmune myelopathies. These include myelopathies associated with myelin oligodendrocyte glycoprotein (MOG) antibodies, anti-aquaporin 4 antibody neuromyelitis optica spectrum disorder (NMO-SD) myelopathies related to systemic lupus erythematosus (SLE), paraneoplastic autoimmune myelopathies, postinfectious autoimmune myelopathies [acute disseminated encephalomyelitis (ADEM)], and myelopathies thought to be immune related [such as multiple sclerosis (MS) and spinal cord sarcoidosis].

The location, size, and enhancement characteristics of the lesion's enhancement assist to narrow down the differential diagnosis, and hence magnetic resonance imaging (MRI) of the spine is essential for the diagnosis.

The classification of these myelopathies has been made easier by the recent finding of several unique, neurospecific autoantibodies that accompany autoimmune myelopathies. These autoantibodies include a cytotoxic T-cell-mediated autoimmune response protein [collapsin response mediator protein 5 (CRMP-5)] causing myelopathy which could be pathogenic (e.g., AQP-4 IgG) or nonpathogenic.

The existence of autoantibodies aids in the diagnosis of cancer, and helps determine the course and effectiveness of treatment, and drives the search for the disease. The first objective whenever a paraneoplastic myelopathy is found would be to find and treat the underlying cancer. The aim of immunotherapy in these autoimmune myelopathies would be to sustain the benefits with a minimum of side effects and maximizing reversibility.

Autoimmune Visual Loss

Numerous autoimmune diseases can impair vision, and they do so through various mechanisms that disrupt the visual pathway.

In autoimmune disorders, the retina, optic nerve, and chiasma can be involved. One of the most frequent causes of vision loss is MS, however, the exact origin of this inflammation in MS is yet unknown.

Aquaporin 4 and MOG are two antibodies that have been linked to the autoimmune disease causing optic neuritis. Optic neuritis (ON) requiring long-term immunosuppression is known as chronic relapsing inflammatory optic neuropathy (CRION).

Apart from postinfective and postvaccinal ON and SLE, which are autoimmune other vasculitides affect the optic nerve either directly or through occlusive vasculopathy. Sarcoidosis affects the optic nerves, but the mechanisms are not clear and could include autoimmunity.

A candidate autoantibody (recoverin) has been described in cancer-associated retinopathy. Visual loss in autoimmune disorders is an expanding area and significant advances in research have resulted in educated guesses on possible molecular targets of autoimmune attack.

AUTOIMMUNE AQP4 CHANNELOPATHIES AND NEUROMYELITIS OPTICA SPECTRUM DISORDERS

A pathogenic autoantibody specific for the AQP4 water channel characterizes neuromyelitis optica spectrum disorders (NMOSD), an emerging discipline. NMO is now understood to be a recurrent disease that affects not just the spinal cord and optic nerves, but also the brain and skeletal muscle.

The circumventricular organs, which cause intractable nausea and vomiting, and the diencephalon, which causes sleep disorders, endocrinopathies, and syndrome of inappropriate antidiuretic hormone secretion (SIADH), are examples of AQP4-enriched locations where NMOSD characteristic lesions occur. The diagnostic criteria for NMOSD are regularly being revised as a result of developments in our understanding of the immunobiology of AQP4 autoimmunity.

Detecting pathogenic AQP4 Ig G extracellular epitopes holds prognostic promise. NMOSD is also referred to as autoimmune AQP-4 channelopathy and the therapeutic options are likely to increase with better understanding of the molecular pathogenesis **(Figs. 2A to D)**.

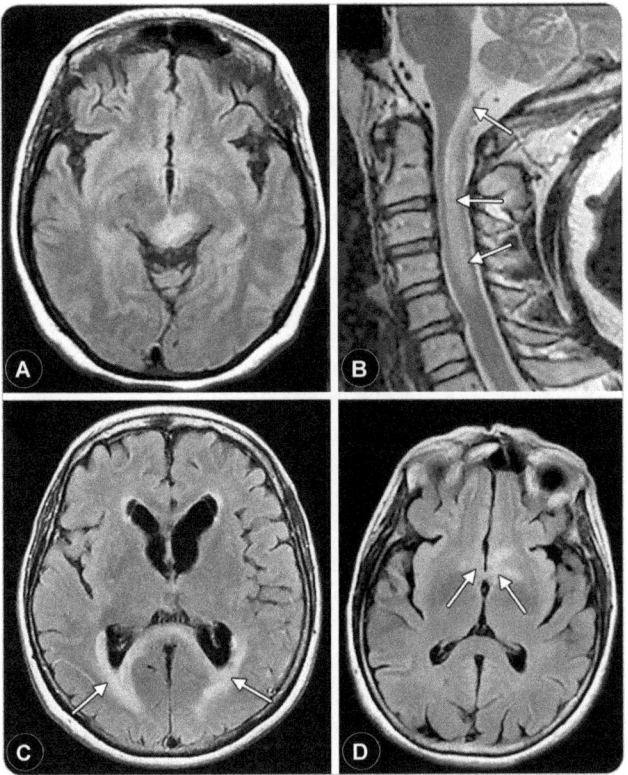

FIG. 2A TO D: In NMOSD MRI axial FLAIR shows hyperintensities in periaqueductal region (A); LETM extending into medulla (B); periependymal region (C); and hypothalamus (D).
(FLAIR: fluid-attenuated inversion recovery; MRI: magnetic resonance imaging; NMOSD: neuromyelitis optica spectrum disorders)

MOG Antibody-associated Disorders

Myelin oligodendrocyte glycoprotein (MOG) is found in the outermost surface of myelin sheaths. MOG antibodies have been found to be present in a subset of patients with ADEM, NMOSD, monophasic, and recurrent ON, and transverse myelitis (TM). MOG antibodies are also present in demyelinating syndromes overlapping with anti-NMDA receptor encephalitis, and with glycine receptor alpha-1 subunit antibody associated optic neuritis. Cell-based assays expressed in human cells using immunofluorescence or fluorescence-activated cell sorting is the preferred way of testing MOG antibodies. During an acute attack intravenous methylprednisolone is used as in other inflammatory demyelinating disorders. Though relapses are common with MOG antibody-associated disorders (MOGAAD), only 40% continue to receive maintenance immunosuppression. Azathioprine, mycophenolate mofetil, and rituximab are commonly used as immunosuppressants to prevent relapse, out of which, rituximab is the most effective.

AUTOIMMUNE AUTONOMIC DISORDERS

The sympathetic and parasympathetic ganglia, enteric ganglia, autonomic nerves, or central autonomic circuits can all be targets of the immune response. Autonomic failure, which may be localized or widespread, is a symptom of autoimmune diseases of the peripheral nervous system. Autonomic hyperactivity is a symptom of autoimmune diseases of the CNS.

Autonomic disorders can be generalized or be limited in their anatomical extent, e.g., isolated gastrointestinal dysmotility. A number of autoantibody biomarkers have been discovered recently, resulting in identification of patients with an autoimmune basis for their autonomic failure or hyperactivity.

Acute autonomic and sensory neuropathy, paraneoplastic autonomic neuropathy, and autoimmune autonomic ganglionopathy (AAG) are examples of peripheral autoimmune autonomic diseases. AAG causes generalized or selective autonomic failure to develop acutely or subacutely. In about 50% of patients of AAG, antibodies against the ganglionic type alpha3 nicotinic acetylcholine receptor (α3AchR) are found.

Some of the disease conditions are seronegative, while others have paraneoplastic antibodies such *ANNA-1* (anti-Hu) that have a significant positive predictive value for malignancy.

Knowing that autonomic disorders have an autoimmune basis may reveal an underlying tumor and allow for treatment using a combination of symptomatic and immunological therapy.

AUTOIMMUNE-MEDIATED PERIPHERAL NEUROPATHIES

- Guillain–Barré syndrome (GBS) or acute inflammatory demyelinating polyneuropathy (AIDP)
- Chronic inflammatory demyelinating polyneuropathy (CIDP)

- CIDP variants
- Multifocal motor neuropathy (MMN)

Systemic Disorder Associated with Immune-Mediated Neuropathies

- Monoclonal gammopathy of unknown significance (MGUS)
- Polyneuropathy, Organomegaly, Endocrinopathy, Monoclonal protein, Skin changes (POEMS) syndrome
- Neuropathy with IgM gammopathy:
  - Waldenstrom macroglobulinemia
  - Mixed cryoglobulinemia
  - Gait ataxia with late-onset polyneuropathy (GALOP)
  - Chronic ataxic neuropathy ophthalmoplegia IgM paraproteinemia, cold agglutinins disialosyl antibodies (CANOMAD) syndrome
- Primary amyloidosis:
  - Other paraneoplastic neuropathies
  - Neuropathy with systemic autoimmune disease
  - Neuropathy with other systemic nonautoimmune diseases

A wide range of symptoms, including subacute progression, asymmetric or multifocal deficits, and specific involvement of motor, sensory, or autonomic nerves are prevalent in autoimmune neuropathies.

Diagnosis becomes difficult because of the overlap of symptoms amongst the various syndromes. History and clinical findings enable a presumptive diagnosis to be made. Apart from tumors, basic laboratory tests are required to rule out metabolic and infectious etiologies. Once these etiologies are ruled out, additional testing with imaging, nerve conduction investigations, and CSF analysis is required. Autoimmune neuropathies can occasionally be paraneoplastic. Antibody testing indicates that the neuropathy may be immune-mediated, but it cannot be considered conclusive.

Indications for Testing

People who exhibit moderate-to-severe sensory and motor symptoms (motor sensory symptomatology) and a progressive course without a known cause may want to undergo autoantibody testing.

Classification: Acute and chronic autoimmune neuropathies are separated into these categories. The GBS and its variants are examples of acute neuropathies. The typical CIDP and its variants are chronic autoimmune neuropathies. The several types of neuropathies include motor, sensory, and combined neuropathies. The antibodies associated with nonparaneoplastic and paraneoplastic neuropathies and their clinical presentations are given in **Tables 1 and 2** below.

TABLE 1: Nonparaneoplastic markers.	
Autoantibody	Examples of associated neuropathic syndrome
GM1	MMN, ALS, GBS, and AMAN
GM2	GBS variants
MAG or SGPG	Inflammatory (often demyelinating) neuropathy with IgM gammopathy, gait ataxia, and hand tremor
Sulfatide	Chronic sensory peripheral neuropathy, GALOP syndrome
GQ1b	Acute ophthalmoplegia, cerebellar ataxia of MFS
GD1b	Sensory peripheral neuropathy MND, GBS
GD1a	Axonal GBS

(ALS: amyotrophic lateral sclerosis; AMAN: acute motor axonal neuropathy; GALOP: gait ataxia late-age onset polyneuropathy; GBS: Guillain–Barré syndrome; MAG: myelin-associated glycoprotein; MFS: Miller Fisher syndrome; MMN: multifocal motor neuropathy; MND: motor neuron disease; SGPG: sulfate-3-glucuronyl paragloboside)

TABLE 2: Paraneoplastic markers.		
Autoantibody	Examples of associated neuropathic syndrome	Associated malignancies
Hu (ANNA-1)	PN, limbic encephalitis, GI dysmotility, ataxia, sensory neuropathy, and autonomic and sensorimotor neuropathies	SCLC
Ri (ANNA-2)	Neuropathy, ataxia, opsoclonus myoclonus	Lung, breast
ANNA-3	Neuropathy, ataxia, limbic encephalopathy	Lung, breast
Amphiphysin	Encephalomyelitis, neuropathy, stiff-person syndrome	Lung, breast
CV2, collapsin response mediator protein 5 (CRMP-5)	PN, limbic encephalitis, ataxia, chorea, optic neuritis	SCLC, thymoma
N-type calcium channel antibodies	PN, other syndromes	Lung, breast

(GI: gastrointestinal; PN: peripheral neuropathy; SCLC: small cell lung cancer)

AUTOIMMUNE NEUROMUSCULAR JUNCTION DISORDERS

Diseases that affect the neuromuscular junction (NMJ) span a broad spectrum. One of the crucial proteins that regulate signaling between the presynaptic nerve ending and the postsynaptic muscular membrane is affected by antibodies, genetic mutations, specific drugs, and toxins in disorders of NMJ.

The most prevalent autoimmune diseases of the NMJ are acquired. Agrin-induced AchR clustering, which is essential for effective neurotransmission, is disrupted by antibodies to AchR or to proteins involved in receptor clustering, especially muscle-specific kinase (MUSK), in people with myasthenia gravis.

Loss of the presynaptic voltage-gated calcium channels causes a reduction in the release of the neurotransmitter acetylcholine in the Lambert–Eaton myasthenic syndrome (LEMS). These diseases are typically identifiable clinically, and serologic tests and electromyography can both corroborate the diagnosis. An accompanying tumor screening would be necessary. For instance, screening for small cell lung cancer in LEMS and thymoma in patients with myasthenia gravis.

Fortunately, there are a variety of symptomatic treatments, immunosuppressive medications, or other immunomodulating therapy available to address these conditions. With the discovery of novel antigens, research is being done to better understand the pathophysiology and make more specialized treatments available.

AUTOIMMUNE MUSCLE DISEASES

Immune-mediated myopathies include polymyositis (PM), dermatomyositis (DM), immune-mediated necrotizing myopathy (IMNM), and inclusion body myositis (IBM) and overlap myositis which includes antisynthetase syndrome.

Elevated muscle enzymes, myopathic electromyographic abnormalities, subacute development of symmetric proximal muscle weakness, and autoantibodies are all present in PM, DM, and IMNM. Their clinical characteristics and histology are used to distinguish them from one another.

Patients with DM can be identified by their cutaneous symptoms. The infiltration of non-necrotic muscle fibers by T cells in PM, perifascicular atrophy in DM, and myofiber necrosis without obvious inflammation in IMNM is distinguishing characteristics on muscle biopsy.

These conditions are categorized as autoimmune disorders, and immunosuppressive medication usually improves the majority of patients' symptoms, if not entirely in dermatomyositis, polymyositis and overlap myositis.

INCLUSION BODY MYOSITIS

Patients with IBM typically exhibit a gradual onset of asymmetric weakness in the proximal quadriceps and the distal muscles (such as wrist flexion). The muscle biopsy reveals rimmed vacuoles with focal lymphocyte infiltration of myofibers. Even though the majority of IBM patients have autoantibodies, immunosuppressive medication does not alter the clinical outcome. The refractory nature of the condition and its progressive course raises the possibility of a myodegenerative component. Recent research suggests that these illnesses constitute a varied family, with each entity including roughly a dozen myositis autoantibodies.

AUTOIMMUNE NEUROLOGIC DISORDERS IN CHILDREN

Children's autoimmune neurologic disorders have significant clinical significance. Childhood antibody-mediated CNS disorders, where the antibodies attach to cell surface epitopes on neuronal or glial proteins, are becoming more well known. Depending on the extent of the brain involvement by the antibodies, the clinical features would be localized or more widespread.

The diseases includes limbic encephalitis and NMDA receptor antibody encephalitis, among many others, and these antibodies may be directed against ion channel receptors and membrane proteins.

Seizures, movement disorders, autonomic dysfunction, and sleep problems, along with distinctive electrophysiologic and neuroimaging findings, may point to a particular antibody-mediated immunological illness. These conditions exhibit phenotypic overlap, and the same condition exhibits phenotypic variation. Immunotherapy significantly improves outcomes, but there is still much scope for improvement.

Immunotherapy

The majority of the data for the treatment of autoimmune neurologic diseases comes from anecdotal reports, large case series, and expert opinion because there have not been many randomized controlled trials (RCTs) in this area. Oncologic therapy and immunotherapy are used to treat autoimmune neurologic diseases.

Improved mechanistic understanding of immunopathology, with a focus on monoclonal antibodies as with myasthenia gravis, NMO, and chronic inflammatory demyelinating polyradiculoneuropathy, is necessary for novel methods, such as novel drug discovery or therapeutic repurposing. Every patient needs a unique treatment strategy and care plan that takes into account their clinical condition, type of antibody, presence or absence of neoplasm, and how they responded to previous therapies.

CHAPTER 11

Movement Disorders

INTRODUCTION

The basal ganglia and cerebellum modulate motor cortical output and allow for smooth coordinated movements. The basal ganglia include the corpus striatum (i.e., the caudate nucleus and putamen), globus pallidus, subthalamic nucleus, substantia nigra, and pedunculopontine nucleus. These are subcortical structures which comprise of groups of gray matter nuclei **(Fig. 1)**.

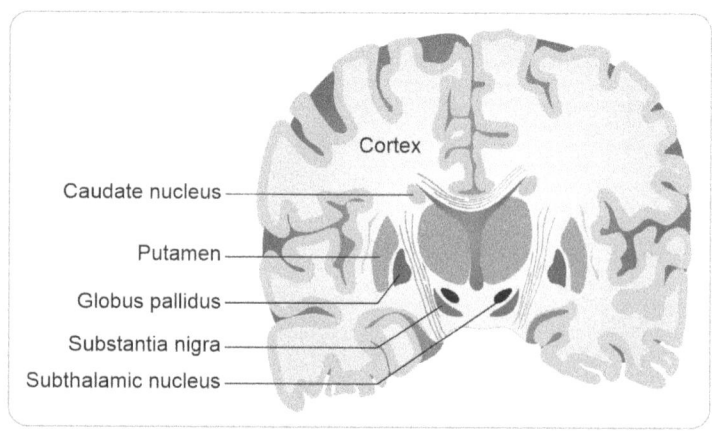

FIG. 1: Anatomy of basal ganglia.

MOVEMENT DISORDERS AND THEIR LOCALIZATION

- Parkinson's disease (PD)—substantia nigra
- Chorea—caudate nucleus
- Dystonia—putamen
- Ballism—subthalamic nucleus
- *Tremors*:
  - Essential tremor (ET)—cerebellum
  - Rubral tremor—red nucleus

Movement disorders can be characterized by impairment of voluntary movements (hypokinetic) or by the presence of involuntary movements (hyperkinetic).

The principal disorder of hypokinesia is "parkinsonism" which refers to several conditions including PD, and other syndromes called "Parkinson plus syndromes" which has parkinsonian features apart from other clinical features.

These Parkinson plus syndromes include Lewy body dementia, MSA, progressive supranuclear palsy (PSP), and corticobasal syndrome (CBS). Parkinsonism can also be caused by medications including antipsychotics such as haloperidol, amisulpride, risperidone, antiemetics like metoclopramide, prokinetic levosulpiride, and calcium channel blockers like cinnarizine and flunarizine.

The four cardinal features of parkinsonism are known by the mnemonic "TRAP":

1. "T" for tremor which in its classical forms is "pill rolling", like someone who is rolling a pill between thumb and index finger.
2. "R" stands for rigidity which is often described as cog wheeling. When an examiner attempts to passively move a limb, there is a series of stops or stalls like a cog on the wheel.

    When a limb is rigid throughout the entire passive movement, it is described as lead-pipe rigidity as it resembles moving a lead pipe.

    Cogwheel and lead-pipe rigidity are distinct from clasp knife spasticity which occurs with corticospinal tract involvement.
3. "A" reflects akinesia which is the absence of movement and is the most severe form of bradykinesia. Slow shuffling gait and a mask-like face are also forms of bradykinesia or reduced movements.

4. "P" stands for postural instability, because of which the patient has a stooped posture with imbalance in walking and is associated with falls.

The symptoms are asymmetric with onset on one side in idiopathic Parkinson's disease (IPD), whereas in other forms of parkinsonism and drug-induced parkinsonism, it is bilateral and symmetric. IPD was first recognized by James Parkinson in 1817.

Parkinson's disease results from accumulation of the protein alpha-synuclein within the neurons of substantia nigra which secretes dopamine. The intracellular inclusion bodies are called Lewy bodies.

Idiopathic PD has its onset in the sixth and seventh decades and accounts for >75% of parkinsonism. There are genetic factors which have a role in the causation of PD. Genetic PD has to be considered in persons with age of onset >45 years and in those with familial occurrence.

The relevant genes involved are:
- Alpha synuclein gene (*PARK1*)—chromosome 4q; AD inheritance
- Parkin gene (*PARK2*)—chromosome 6q with AR inheritance in sporadic cases. Familial cases of PD can be caused by mutations in the *LRRK*, *PARK7*, *PINK1*, *PRKN*, or *SNCA* gene or by alterations in genes yet to be identified. Mutations in some of these genes may also play a role in cases that appear to be sporadic.

A couple of decades ago, no genetic connection was linked to PD. However, in the past 2 decades, 26 new genetic variants associated with PD have been identified by genome-wide association studies or GWAS.

Currently testing is available for the following genes:
- *GBA*, *PARK7*, *SNCA*, *LRRK2*, *PARKIN*, and *PINK1*
- Leucine-rich repeat kinase 2 *(LRRK2)*, also known as dardarin and *PARK8*, a kinase enzyme that in humans is encoded by the *LRRK2* gene.

However, the vast majority of PD is genetically complex and it is caused by the combined action of common genetic variants in concert with environmental factors. These show only moderate effects on PD risk. Most cases of PD probably result from a complex interaction of genetic and environmental factors as mentioned above. These cases are classified as sporadic and occur in people with no family history and the cause of these sporadic cases is unclear. Approximately 15% of people with PD have a family history of this disorder. Familial cases are caused by the mutation in the genes mentioned above (*LRRK, PARK7, PINK1, PRKN,* and *SNCA* genes). Alteration in certain genes *GBA* and *UCHC1* does not cause PD. *LRRK2* and *SNCA* follow autosomal dominant pattern. *PARK7, PINK1,* or *PRKN* follows autosomal recessive pattern.

Parkinson's disease worsens over time and differs in severity in different individuals. Not all people who have PD will have all the manifestations and the rate of progression differs in different individuals.

Hoehn and Yahr scale which classifies the disease into five stages was used to categorize the patients—stage 1 and stage 2 are considered—mild; stage 3 is considered moderate, and stage 4 and stage 5 are considered severe.

1. *Stage 1*: Mild unilateral involvement—tremor, rigidity, clumsy leg, with reduced expression on one side of the face.
2. *Stage 2*: Mild bilateral and midline with
    i. Decreased facial expression, decreased blinking
    ii. Speech abnormalities, trunk muscle rigidity
3. *Stage 3*: Moderate characterized by loss of balance and slowness of movements.
    i. Balance is compromised.
    ii. It cannot make quick adjustments in movements.
    iii. Almost all symptoms are present.
4. *Stage 4*: Severe
    i. Symptoms disabling
    ii. It may be able to walk and stand but incapacitated.
    iii. Patient is unable to live an independent life and needs assistance.
5. *Stage 5*: Severe
    i. Symptoms of PD are severe and are characterized by an inability to rise from bed independently.
    ii. Patients fall when standing or turning.
    iii. May freeze or stumble when walking
    iv. Have hallucinations or delusions which could also be due to the medications

Stage 1 and 2: Early PD
Stage 3: Mild PD
Stage 4 and 5: Advanced PD

Unified Parkinson Disease Rating Scale (UPDRS) and the Movement Disorder Society (MDS)-UPDRS are a comprehensive 50 question assessment of both motor and nonmotor symptoms associated with PD.

PARKINSON'S DISEASE SYMPTOMS

The major symptoms are:
- Bradykinesia (slowness of movement)
- Rigidity (muscle stiffness)
- Stooped posture
- Freezing (experiencing a sudden inability to move)
- Tremor (shaking)
- Micrographia (small handwriting)
- Shuffling gait
- Fatigue
- Apathy
- Loss of sense of smell (hyposmia and anosmia)
- Sleep disturbance
- Constipation
- Depression
- Micturition difficulty

Possible etiology includes:
- Idiopathic
- Pesticides, toxins, and chemicals
- Head trauma
- Genetic factors

TREATMENT OF PARKINSON'S DISEASE

- Medications
- Deep brain stimulation (DBS), MR guided focused ultrasound (MRgFUS)
- Multidisciplinary therapy (counselors, nurses, and allied health professionals)

Medications

Parkinson's disease is due to deficiency of the neurotransmitter dopamine.

The goal of medication therapy is to increase dopamine levels in the brain. Most of the medications come under one of the following categories:
- *Levodopa* replaces dopamine.
- *Dopamine agonists*—dopamine mimicker
- *COMT (catechol-O-methyltransferase) inhibitors (entacapone)* which is used along with levodopa. Levodopa is not broken

down in the intestine due to inhibition of the COMT enzyme, by this inhibitor, which increases the amount of dopamine reaching the brain.
- *Anticholinergics* block the effect of acetylcholine, to enable it to balance its level with dopamine.
- *Amantadine* is a noncompetitive antagonist of N-methyl-D-aspartate (NMDA) receptor and improves dopamine transmission by increasing dopamine release and reducing its reuptake.
- *Monoamine oxidase (MAO) type B inhibitors* slow down the metabolism of dopamine in the brain making, dopamine available for a longer time.
- *Carbidopa* inhibits peripheral metabolism of levodopa by acting as dopa decarboxylase inhibitor reducing the conversion of levodopa to dopamine in blood stream prematurely before getting into the brain, enabling smaller doses of levodopa to be effective.
- *Carbidopa/levodopa* remains the most effective drug to treat PD. Medication can help with symptom relief, but does not stop the disease progression over time. Dopa may lose its effectiveness with time, and an increase in dosage could cause unwanted side effects, dyskinesias.

Surgical Option

Surgery is an option, but is not suited for everyone and candidates will have to be meticulously selected. Only IPD patients improve and tremor is the symptom which improves most, and rigidity and bradykinesia improve to a lesser extent. Presence of dementia or psychosis is a contraindication for surgery.

Deep brain stimulation of the subthalamic nuclei (STN) is the most effective surgical treatment and gives good relief for tremors. DBS of the globus pallidus interna (GPi) is also equally effective and is being done in several centers and is the preferred site now.

Focussed ultrasound ablation of the thalamic nucleus and pallidothalamic tractotomy is gaining traction as an alternative to the invasive DBS. It should be understood that neither DBS nor MRgFUS provides a cure for Parkinson's disease and at best only ameliorates the symptom of tremors and to a lesser extent rigidity and bradykinesia.

Exercise

Regular exercise helps lessen PD symptoms and enhance overall quality of life. Dancing, tai chi, yoga, swimming, cycling, apart from walking, are quality exercises for Parkinson patients.

SECONDARY PARKINSONISM

When symptoms of PD are brought on by identifiable causes, such as infections, trauma, vascular assaults, metabolic disorders, toxins, and drugs, it is called secondary parkinsonism.
They include:
- Brain injury
- Stroke
- Encephalitis, meningitis, and human immunodeficiency virus/acquired immunodeficiency syndrome (HIV/AIDS)
- Wilson's disease (WD) neurodegeneration with brain iron accumulation (NBIA).
- *Medications*: Antipsychotics, levosulpiride, metoclopramide, and calcium channel antagonists cinnarizine and flunarizine
- Carbon monoxide and mercury poisoning
- 1-methyl-4-phenyl-1,2,3,6-tetrahydropyridine (MPTP) contaminant in street drugs

As many causes of secondary parkinsonism also lead to cognitive impairment of varying severity, confusion and memory impairment could also occur.

Treatment

If the condition is considered to be due to medications, the medicines will have to be stopped. Treatment of underlying causes such as infections and stroke will reduce the symptoms and prevent worsening. Dopamine can be administered but the improvement, if at all, is likely to be less than in IPD.

ATYPICAL PARKINSONIAN DISORDER

Atypical Parkinsonian disorders are progressive conditions that share some of the hallmarks of PD but do not improve with levodopa therapy. They are linked to an aberrant protein buildup within brain cells. The word describes a number of ailments that affect only certain parts of the brain and have a characteristic progression.

- *Dementia with Lewy bodies disease (DLBD)* is due to an abnormal accumulation of alpha-synuclein protein in the neurons and clinical features of cognitive impairment, fluctuating attention, and visual hallucinations which exacerbate on taking antipsychotics. Other manifestations include extrapyramidal features and daytime sleep of 2 hours or more.
- *Progressive supranuclear palsy* is a tauopathy, affecting the substantia nigra, brainstem, cerebellum, and frontal lobes. Parkinsonian features with axial rigidity, and falls early in the course of disease are the key features. The characteristic sign is supranuclear vertical gaze palsy. Tremors are not a prominent feature **(Figs. 2 to 4)**.

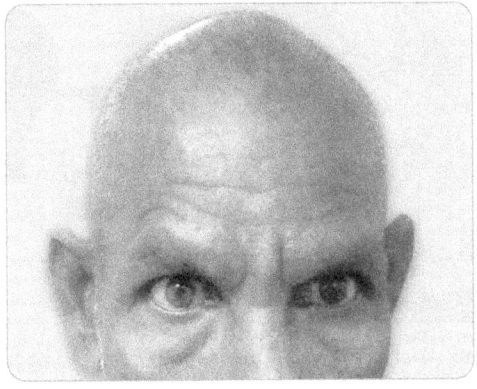

FIG. 2: Vertical wrinkles in the glabella region and bridge of the nose is known as procerus sign, which is seen in progressive supranuclear palsy (PSP), due to contraction of the procerus muscle.

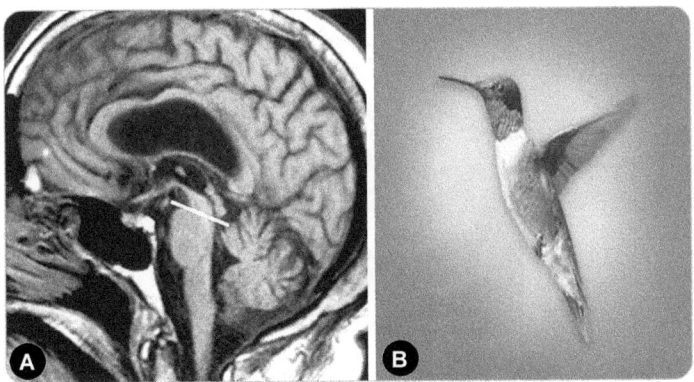

FIGS. 3A AND B: T1 sagittal magnetic resonance imaging (MRI) brain showing midbrain atrophy with preserved pons mimicking a hummingbird.

- *Multiple system atrophy (MSA)*: Another synucleinopathy that affects the cerebellum, substantia nigra, and the autonomic nervous system. Light headedness on standing (orthostasis) with fall of standing BP, urinary urgency, retention, incontinence, erectile dysfunction, and constipation are the autonomic symptoms which predominate early in the disease course. MSA can affect the cerebellum with gait ataxia and appendicular ataxia known as MSA-cerebellar type (MSA-C). When Parkinsonian features predominate, it is designated MSA-parkinsonism (MSA-P) **(Figs. 5 and 6)**.

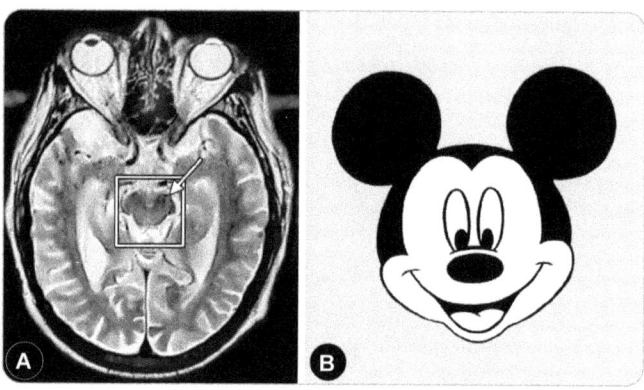

FIGS. 4A AND B: Axial T2-weighted magnetic resonance imaging (MRI) of the brain showing selective atrophy of the midbrain tegmentum with relative preservation of tectum and cerebral peduncles resembling the head of Mickey mouse.

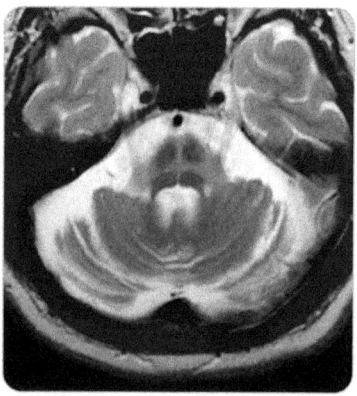

FIG. 5: Magnetic resonance imaging (MRI) brain with T2 hyperintensity forming a cross on axial images, due to selective degeneration of pontocerebellar tracts as seen in multiple system atrophy-cerebellar type (MSA-C).

- *Corticobasal syndrome* is a rare tauopathy, which affects one-half of the body with myoclonus and dystonia. One of the main characteristics of CBS is apraxia, which is the inability to exhibit or recognize the use of everyday things. A pathognomonic sign of CBS is the "alien limb phenomenon," in which the patient perceives his or her limb as a foreign entity and is unable to regulate its movements **(Fig. 7)**.

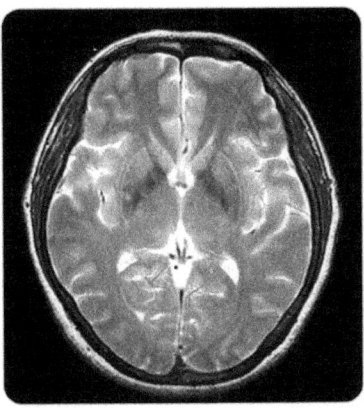

FIG. 6: Magnetic resonance imaging (MRI) brain T2 axial view showing linear hyperintensity surrounding the putamen known as putaminal rim sign as seen in multiple system atrophy-parkinsonism (MSA–P).

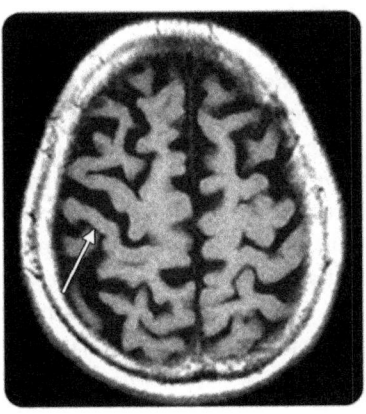

FIG. 7: Asymmetric frontoparietal cortical atrophy with an emphasis on the central region in a T1-weighted axial section MRI is seen in corticobasal ganglionic degeneration.

Atypical parkinsonian disorders are not considered to be genetic currently. Most are due to unknown etiology though long-term drug exposure and trauma could be the causes in some. Though characteristic imaging features have been described in PSP and MSA, the changes appear quite late in the course of the disease and are hence not helpful in the early phases.

Since there are currently no imaging, biochemical, or genetic abnormalities that can definitively identify or differentiate between these many conditions, the diagnosis of parkinsonian syndromes is solely clinical.

Clinical experience has a significant impact on diagnostic accuracy, and even among movement disorder specialists, the clinical diagnosis might alter over time as new clinical signs appear. Dopamine transporter (DAT) scan can identify Parkinsonian disorders but cannot differentiate PD from atypical parkinsonism as it is abnormal in all of these.

Vascular Parkinsonism

Vascular parkinsonism is suspected when the person has lower limb involvement with relative sparing of upper limbs, upper trunk, and facial expressions with predominant gait dysfunction. Only less than half the number of patients show pyramidal signs, which when present, exclude PD. MRI of the brain shows extensive white matter lesions in most cases.

Key points of Parkinsonian syndromes are:
- Bradykinesia, a clinical symptom that must always be present to classify parkinsonism as a syndrome.
- A progressive decrease in movement amplitude or speed is necessary to diagnose bradykinesia as PD. However, in PSP, slower movements without decrement (hypokinesia) may be the only indication of basal ganglia impairment.
- Rigidity, which refers to an excessive increase in resistance to passive movements which is velocity independent.
- Slowly pronating and supinating the forearms can generally lessen PD tremors while enhancing dystonic tremors.
- Parkinson's disease patients' gaits tend to stutter or freeze more noticeably when turning or passing through tight places, such doorways.
- Postural instability characterized by falls within 2 years of onset of symptoms is indicative of an atypical parkinsonism disorder as falls are usually a late occurrence in idiopathic PD (IPD).

- Parkinson's disease onset at a younger age is linked to longer survival and a slower progression of disability.
- Dyskinesia are caused by dopamine agonists and MAO inhibitors, used along with the dopa although it happens with levodopa alone in high doses.
- A poor response to levodopa, early postural instability with falls, early executive dysfunction, slowing of vertical saccades and supranuclear vertical gaze paresis, or early dysarthria or dysphagia, is diagnostic of progressive supranuclear palsy (PSP).
- Pure akinesia with freezing and absence of limb rigidity are significant manifestations of PSP.
- Progressive and severe autonomic dysfunction, which frequently predominates the early clinical picture and occurs up to several years before the emergence of motor symptoms, is inevitably linked to MSA.
- In MSA-P, action, spontaneous, and stimulus-sensitive distal myoclonus occurs more frequently than rest tremor.
- When midodrine is ineffective, other medications such as indomethacin or pyridostigmine may be used to treat orthostatic hypotension.
- Corticobasal syndrome is characterized by an asymmetric, progressive parkinsonism with ideomotor apraxia, rigidity, myoclonus, and dystonia that is frequently accompanied by an alien limb phenomenon. Various pathologies, such as corticobasal degeneration (CBD) and PSP, frontotemporal lobar degeneration (FTLD), and Alzheimer's disease can cause clinical features of CBS and are included under the rubric of CBS.
- Two out of the following three features must be present asymmetrically to meet the criteria for likely CBD.
  1. limb dystonia
  2. Limb rigidity or akinesia
  3. Limb myoclonus and two of the following:
     i. Limb or orobuccal apraxia
     ii. Alien limb phenomenon
     iii. Cortical sensory deficit

Pyramidal symptoms rule out PD and support the diagnosis of vascular parkinsonism. The various parkinsonian syndromes can be distinguished by their subtle but distinct signs and symptoms, which can be recognized by careful examination.

The establishment of appropriate therapy guided by a conclusive diagnosis that benefits the patients and their carers may result from taking into consideration the distinctions, notably in the manner of presentation and progression of the illness.

As disease-specific treatment emerges distinctive diagnosis of the different syndromes will become increasingly important.

Distinguishing SWEDD (scans without evidence for dopaminergic deficit) patients with asymmetric resting tremor from Parkinson's is accomplished by doing a 99^mTc-TRODAT-1 single-photon emission computed tomography (SPECT) scan.

Even in the absence of Lewy body neurodegeneration, patients with segmental dystonia might have asymmetric slow movements and rest tremor. When the clinical signs advance, it does so very slowly and rarely necessitates the use of drugs. In this case, the TRODAT SPECT scan indicated above can help distinguish between this condition and PD tremor. The scan is abnormal only in parkinsonism.

Presence of hypokinesia, with no progressive decrement of movement amplitude, position specific tremor, and dystonia in the same limb would be suggestive of dystonic tremor rather than PD tremor.

In parkinsonism and frontotemporal dementia (FTD), the clinical features overlap. FTD syndrome patients can have signs and symptoms of parkinsonism, before, during, or after the occurrence of frontal cognitive or behavioral disturbances.

The spectrum of FTD comprises of the behavioral variant, the semantic variant, and FTD—amyotrophic lateral sclerosis (ALS) types.

These phenotypes can be sporadic:
- Namely the tauopathies—CBD and PSP
- The *TARDNA*-binding protein-43 (*TDP-43* proteinopathies with or without ALS are familial)
- Proteinopathies due to progranulin or *C9ORF72* mutations
- FTD with parkinsonism linked to chromosome 17

Classic PSP shows symmetric parkinsonism and brainstem predominant atrophic features.

Classic CBD presents with markedly asymmetric parkinsonism with predominant cortical atrophy.

The FTLD spectrum includes the less common cooccurrence of behavioral or personality changes, bulbar, or pseudobulbar features, and these features would be classified as FTLD-tau when PSP-like features are associated and FTLD-TDP when CBS features or language abnormalities are associated.

The clinical signs which help in the differential diagnosis of hypokinetic disorders are:
- *Tremors which can be*:
  - Rest tremors in IPD or dystonic tremor
  - Postural and resting tremor in PD, Fragile X tremor ataxia syndrome (FXTAS)
  - Coarse postural and action tremor in WD, and MSA
- Autonomic symptoms present in MSA and FXTAS.
- Postural instability, which occurs early in the course of the disease in PSP and MSA and late in PD.
- Cerebellar features, both appendicular and gait ataxias seen in MSA, WD, spinocerebellar ataxia (SCA), and PSP-C.
- Pyramidal signs seen in MSA, WD, and vascular parkinsonism.
- Cognitive or behavioral changes which occur with FTD, and the syndromes of parkinsonism DLBD, PSP, PDD (Parkinson disease dementia) and WD.

There is usually only minimal or no cognitive involvement in MSA.
- Dystonic posturing in various forms as under:
  - Blepharospasms, facial dystonia in PSP
  - Orofacial dystonias seen in MSA and with dopaminergic drugs, neurometabolic disorders such as WD and Huntington's disease (HD).
  - Lower limb dystonia in juvenile PD, Dopa responsive dystonia (DRD), WD, and rapid-onset dystonia parkinsonism.
  - Limb dystonia associated with useless hand in possible CBS
  - Truncal dystonia/camptocormia/Pisa sign associated with MSA
- Myoclonus, seen in CBS, Creutzfeldt–Jakob disease (CJD), and autoimmune encephalopathy
- Stridor, suggesting MSA, and IgLON5 encephalopathy
- Pseudobulbar features with dysarthria and dysphagia, in PSP, vascular parkinsonism, MSA, and WD
- Hallucinations seen in DLBD, medication induced in IPD, and are not common in MSA.
- Neuropsychiatric manifestations in WD, DLBD, HD, and juvenile PD
- REM sleep behavior disorders (RBD) in synucleinopathies namely IPD, MSA, and DLBD
- Excessive daytime sleepiness occurs in MSA, DLBD, and with medication-induced hypokinesia.

- Sleep, which benefits patients with DRD and autosomal recessive young onset Parkinson disease (YOPD)
- Ocular findings and loss of sense of smell

The following are the disorders which need to be considered in relation to the loss of sense of smell and the various ocular findings:
- Anosmia—IPD and DLBD
- Retinitis pigmentosa—pantothenate kinase-associated neurodegeneration (PKAN)
- Impaired convergence—MSA
- Vertical gaze paresis—PSP
- Oculomotor apraxia and apraxia of eyelid opening—PSP
- Square wave jerks in the eyes—PSP
- Gunslinger's gait with recurrent falls in erect posture and decreased arm swing in PSP
- Rocket sign, i.e., getting up from the chair quickly and then falling back because of postural instability in PSP

HYPERKINETIC MOVEMENT DISORDERS

Hyperkinesia refers to increased muscle activity resulting in excessive abnormal movements or excess of normal movements.

Many of the hyperkinetic movements are the result of improper regulation of the basal ganglia—thalamocortical circuitry. Overactivity of the direct excitatory pathway combined with decreased activity of the inhibitory indirect pathway results in the activation of the thalamic neurons and excitation of cortical neurons resulting in increased motor output. Another feature of hyperkinetic disorders or hyperkinesia is that they are associated with hypotonia or decreased muscle tone. Quite a number of hyperkinetic disorders are psychological in nature and are often present in childhood. Descriptions used in relation to specific movements help in identifying a disorder and should include the following details regarding the movement noted in a state when the body movement is minimal that is on maintaining a posture.

The following terms are used to describe the movements:
- A discrete movement is one, wherein a new posture is adopted without any other posture intruding and interrupting the process.
- Rhythmic movements are those which occur in cycles of the same movements.

- Repetitive, recurrent, and reciprocal movements describe a movement of body or joint position, which occur more than once, though not necessarily in a cyclic manner.
- Overflow movement refers to unwanted movement that occurs in addition to desired movement. It is usually associated with dystonic movements due to an inability to suppress the unwanted muscle movement.

While evaluating these movements the following points also need to be considered:
- The frequency of occurrence
- Whether they can be suppressed by the patients will or, with sensory tricks (geste antagoniste) or, by restraint
- Awareness of the movement by the individual while it is occurring.
- The urge or desire to make the movement
- Whether the movement is triggered at rest, or during an action, or during a specific task.

The common hyperkinetic movements are tremor, chorea, dystonia, tics, myoclonus, ballism, and stereotypies.

Tremor

Tremor is a rhythmic, back-and-forth oscillatory involuntary movement occurring at a joint with symmetric velocity in both directions. It frequently results from the rhythmic alternate contraction of agonist and antagonist muscles, but not always. According to the state in which tremor is maximal, it is classified as either rest tremor, postural tremor, or action tremor.

Intention tremor is a distinct type of tremor that is linked to cerebellar dysfunction. It is characterized by the tremor getting worse as the limb approaches the goal and is brought on by erroneous movements that overshoot and overcorrect.

Dystonia

It is a condition of movement in which twisting and repetitive movements, abnormal postures, or both are brought on by involuntary, sustained or intermittent, and muscle contractions.

Dystonic postures are usually repeated, with a particular posture or with characteristic patterns. Foot inversion, ulnar deviation at the wrist, or lordotic trunk postures are the common dystonic postures in children.

These postures may be sustained or occur for very brief periods. Dystonic movements usually occur on voluntary movement, or on assuming a particular body posture, or on specific tasks. Dystonic movements are not present in sleep. Though cocontraction is a feature of dystonia, it is not necessary to maintain a stable or dystonic posture.

Damage to the putamen, globus pallidus, and basal ganglia is associated with dystonia. However, no basal ganglia lesion is found in many dystonia instances, and recent research indicates that the cerebellum, brainstem, or sensory cortex may also be involved.

Chorea

These movements appear randomly and each movement has a distinct start and end point, though often it is difficult to identify these as one flows on to the other. Choreic movements are more rapid than dystonic movements and are unpredictable. "Parakinesia" is the term applied to the involuntary movement which is made to look like a purposeful movement in an attempt to mask the involuntary movements.

The individual movement fragments in chorea can be identified as brief and jerky, whereas in athetosis the movements are not discrete and is a sinuous, continuously flowing random movement.

Chorea lacks the rhythmicity and predictability of tremor and differs from myoclonus in that, only some choreic movements are quick while in myoclonus all movements are quick. Myoclonus is also more stereotyped. Chorea differs from tics in that choreic movements cannot be suppressed voluntarily, whereas tics can be suppressed.

Ballism is chorea that affects the proximal parts such as the shoulder and hip, because of which, the movements of the limbs are of large amplitude with a flinging quality. Chorea can be due to disorders of the thalamus, cerebral cortex, cerebellum, basal ganglia, and as mentioned earlier.

The phenomenology depends on the cause and the site of manifestation, e.g., poststreptococcal infection-associated chorea, known as Sydenham's chorea, is distal, with piano playing movements at the metacarpophalangeal joints of both hands

Encephalitis affects gray matter resulting in chorea and myoclonus that involve proximal and distal muscles of the limbs, neck, trunk, and face. Lesions in the subthalamic nucleus are related with chorea and ballism. A number of genetic and metabolic disorders such as hyperthyroidism, WD, and medication toxicity can cause chorea.

Athetosis is not considered by many to be a separate entity as it very often merges into dystonia. Athetosis is a slow, continuous writhing movement that occurs involuntarily and impairs the maintenance of a steady posture. More so than the proximal portions of the limbs, athetosis affects the distal extremities, such as the hands or feet, but it can also affect the face, neck, and trunk. Athetosis rarely occurs alone; it frequently cooccurs with chorea and dystonia. Choreoathetosis, a mix of chorea and athetosis, is most frequently seen in cerebral palsy and kernicterus **(Fig. 8)**.

Severe sensory loss in the distal limbs as in sensory ganglionopathy of diabetes mellitus or paraneoplastic etiology can cause athetosis like movements termed as "pseudoathetosis".

Myoclonus

Myoclonus is a brief, shock-like jerk occurring due to sudden involuntary contraction or relaxation of one or more muscles occurring in sequence.

Myoclonus can be:
- *Synchronous*: When several muscles are simultaneously contracting.

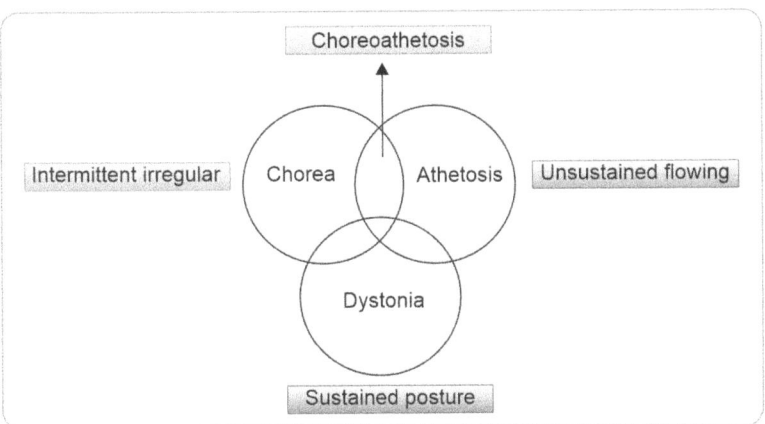

FIG. 8: Co-occurrence of hyperkinetic movement disorders namely chorea, dystonia and athetosis.

- *Asynchronous*: When several muscles are contracting at different times.
- *Multifocal*: When more than one muscle is affected at random.
- *Generalized*: When many muscles are involved simultaneously.
- *Positive myoclonus*: Characterized by sudden muscle contraction resulting in a unidirectional movement
- *Negative myoclonus*: Sudden muscle relaxation with interruption of muscle activity

Myoclonus can be:
- Action myoclonus
- Postural myoclonus
- Rest myoclonus

The sites of origin are:
- Cortical
- Subcortical
- Brainstem
- Propriospinal and spinal

The involvement of the pharyngeal musculature causes palatal myoclonus and because of the rhythmicity of these movements, it is also called palatal tremor.

Asynchronous multifocal myoclonus may be difficult to differentiate from chorea but the more complex and often slow fragments can help identify choreiform movements.

Myoclonus is often seen in gray matter neurodegenerative disease, progressive myoclonic epilepsy in children, metabolic disorders, tumors, infection, and could be associated with seizures, delirium or dementia as seen in CJD and CBS, and hypoxic encephalopathy.

Tics

These are repetitive, intermittent movements, or parts of movements which can be suppressed voluntarily. There is an urge to perform the movement, and such movements are referred to as unvoluntary.

This movement is predictable, and can be brought on by stress, suggestion, and excitement. Generally, tics do not cause injury, though self-injurious tics do occur in 10–15% of Tourette syndrome. The intervening periods of normalcy without tics are a defining trait of tics.

Tics can be classified as:
- Simple motor tics which is a single brief stereotyped movement.
- Complex motor tics which are more complex or sequential movements involving multiple muscle groups.
- Phonic tics which are characterized by simple brief phonation or vocalization. It is important to realize that tics have a high association with obsessive compulsive disorder which makes it difficult to differentiate from complex motor tics.
- Tics may wax and wane for several months to years, and the movements may be different at different times, while some disappear completely. Sustained posture can be a form of tic when it is called "dystonic tic". Similarly, tic can manifest as a sudden jerky or shock-like movement when it is termed "myoclonic tics".

These movements do not share a common pathophysiology with either dystonia or myoclonus. Voluntary movements are not interfered by tics whereas dystonia interferes.

Only rarely are tics pathological, being associated with degenerative or inflammatory diseases of the basal ganglia when they are part of a complex of involuntary movements (complex movement disorder).

Stereotypies

Stereotypies are repetitive movements that can be voluntarily suppressed. The movements are most often rhythmic and involves fingers and wrists and more proximal parts of the upper limbs. The lower limbs are seldom affected, and are often bilateral, in the form of waving or flapping of the hands or arms. The ability to suppress the movements voluntarily distinguishes them from tremor or myoclonus.

The lack of a premonitory urge differentiates stereotypy from a tic, but the subject should be cognizant enough to know that there is no premonitory urge when asked about it.

Stereotypies are common in healthy children though they are a well-known accompaniment of developmental syndromes including autism spectrum disorders. The presence of stereotypy by itself does not suggest a neurological disorder.

Key Features of Hyperkinetic Disorders

Key features of hyperkinetic disorders are given in **Table 1**.

TABLE 1: Key features of hyperkinetic disorders.

Movement	Rhythmic	Suppressible	Repeated posture	Repeated stereotyped movement
Myoclonus	Sometimes	No	Sometimes	Usually
Tics	No	Usually yes	Yes	Yes
Athetosis	No	No	No	No
Dystonia	Rarely	Partial or briefly	Yes	Sometimes
Tremor	Yes	Sometimes briefly	No	Yes
Chorea	No	No	No	Rarely
Stereotypies	Yes	Yes	Sometimes	Yes

ELECTROPHYSIOLOGICAL STUDIES IN HYPERKINETIC MOVEMENTS

The motor unit recruitment is normal but overflow of muscle activity from nearby muscles does occur with dystonia. Myoclonus shows brief rhythmic bursts or pauses of electromyography (EMG) activity. Enlarged SSEP (somatosensory evoked potential) and increased long-latency reflexes are found in myoclonus of cortical origin.

In most cases of tremors, there are alternating bursts in the antagonists and agonists with, at times, synchronous contractions of agonists and antagonists. The EMG in tics and stereotypies resemble voluntary movement though there are only a few studies which have been done.

Less Common Hyperkinesias

These include abdominal dyskinesia, akathisia, hemifacial spasm, hyperekplexia (startle syndromes) "jumpy stumps", painful moving toes and fingers, myokymia, synkinesis, myorhythmia, and paroxysmal dyskinesia.

Hyperkinetic movement disorders are diagnosed clinically and the underlying metabolic, endocrine, immunologic, and toxic causes excluded by blood and cerebrospinal fluid (CSF) work up and where necessary, by genetic studies.

Genetic testing and paraneoplastic panels may be needed for select cases. Imaging will help identify characteristic features

of certain movement disorders and their underlying structural abnormality.
- *Structural abnormalities* of stroke and tumors can be associated with dystonia or ballism.
- *Demyelinating lesions* may be seen in patients with dystonia and ataxia.
- *Vasculitic* features are noted as cause of chorea.
- *Anoxic change* is associated with widespread or multifocal myoclonus.

In all of the above situations, brain MRI and, for spinal, propriospinal myoclonus, and abdominal dyskinesias, spine MRI are done, to exclude structural abnormalities.

Dopamine transporter SPECT scan may be useful in differentiating ET and dystonic tremor from PD tremor and also in distinguish dopamine responsive dystonia (DRD) from YOPD. It is also useful for differentiating parkinsonism from its mimics. DAT scan will be abnormal in PD, PSP, MSA, Lewy body dementia, and CBS and will not be able to differentiate one from the other.

Treatment

Botulinum toxin injection is useful for focal dystonia. Anticholinergics, dopaminergics, dopamine depletors, and gamma-aminobutyric acid (GABA) agonists are of variable benefit in these hyperkinetic disorders. Tetrabenazine and valbenazine are helpful in tardive dyskinesia, dystonia, and chorea. Typical and atypical antipsychotics are often used in chorea and for the psychiatric symptomatology, associated with neurodegenerative disorders.

Deep brain stimulation is a treatment option in a variety of hyperkinetic disorders such as tremors, tardive dyskinesia, myoclonus, dystonia, and neuroacanthocytosis-related movements.

CHAPTER 12

Infections of the Nervous System

INTRODUCTION

The five main causative organisms of central nervous system (CNS) infections are:
1. Bacterial
2. Viral
3. Fungal
4. Parasitic
5. Prion proteins

Fungal infection causes meningitis, brain abscess, and spinal epidural abscess. The fungal organisms involved are cryptococcosis, *Candida*, aspergillosis, nocardiosis, and mucormycosis.

Parasitic infections of the CNS include neurocysticercosis, toxoplasmosis, echinococcosis (hydatidosis), primary amoebic meningoencephalitis, and malaria.

Bacterial infections include tuberculosis (TB), leprosy, neurosyphilis, neuroborreliosis, brucellosis, apart from the grampositive and gram-negative organisms causing bacterial meningitides and brain abscess.

A number of viruses are known to affect the brain causing acute encephalitis. The common viruses are the tick-borne viruses (TBV), herpes simplex virus (HSV), dengue, chikungunya, and Japanese B viruses, rabies virus, Varicella-zoster, measles, Nipah, Zika, Ebola, Powassan and COVID-19 viruses all of which could affect the brain.

The slow virus infections include subacute sclerosing pan encephalitis (SSPE) due to measles virus, progressive multifocal leukoencephalopathy (PML) related to John Cunningham (JC) virus, and acquired immunodeficiency syndrome (AIDS) due to human immunodeficiency virus (HIV).

The prion diseases are Creutzfeldt-Jakob disease (CJD), fatal familial insomnia, Gerstmann-Straussler-Scheinker syndrome, and Kuru.

Postinfectious diseases of the nervous system include:
- Pediatric autoimmune neuropsychiatric disorders associated with streptococcal infections (PANDAs)
- Sydenham's chorea
- Acute disseminated encephalomyelitis (ADEM)
- Guillain-Barré syndrome (GBS)

All of which are considered to be postinfective immune-mediated disorders.

ACUTE BACTERIAL MENINGITIS

It is the bacterial infection-induced inflammation of the meninges and the subarachnoid space, which has the potential to be fatal. The clinical features are fever, headache, meningeal signs, and alteration of sensorium, though all patients need not have all of the above features. Elderly (>65 years) can have atypical presentation with only confusion and without headache or neck stiffness or fever. Vasospasm and thrombosis of the arteries, veins, and arterioles can occur in meningitis.

Meningitis can be acquired in the community or in the hospital settings in immune compromised, and in those with chronic illness, or after head trauma or neurosurgical procedures.

Lumbar puncture and cerebrospinal fluid (CSF) examinations are the investigation of choice in confirming the diagnosis and identifying the causative organisms. Lumbar puncture is usually done after a computed tomography (CT) scan of the brain has been done to exclude increased intracranial pressure, caused by structural abnormalities. The most frequent etiological agent of community-acquired bacterial meningitis is streptococcus pneumonia.

A quicker and more accurate diagnosis is made possible by newer technologies such as multiplex polymerase chain reaction (PCR) and those that include proteomics and genetic sequencing. Catridge Based Nucleic Acid Amplification Test (CBNAAT) for

mycobacterium tuberculosis identification. The standard treatment schedule recommended as broad-spectrum treatment for bacterial meningitis includes:
- Ceftriaxone to a maximum of 4 g/day in two doses ±
- Vancomycin 60 mg/kg/day in four divided doses or ampicillin 2 g every 4 hours.

Steroid is given early as an adjunct, and should ideally be commenced with the first dose of the antibiotic. It should be given in high doses of 10 mg of dexamethasone every 4–6 hours initially and then gradually tapered.

Despite appropriate treatment, the complication rate of acute bacterial meningitis is as high as 20%, and the most commonly reported sequelae are hearing loss, cognitive impairment, and epilepsy.

VIRAL MENINGITIS AND VIRAL ENCEPHALITIS

It is essential to differentiate viral meningitis from viral encephalitis as the prognosis differs greatly even though they are caused by the same organism. As an example, Herpes simplex 1 and 2 meningitis may need little or no antiviral treatment, and has no sequelae whereas herpes simplex encephalitis needs high-dose acyclovir treatment for at least 14 days and results in 50% chance of residual sequelae.

In immunocompetent individuals, viral meningitis is frequently benign and self-limited, leaving few long-term effects.

Meningitis can be brought on by a variety of viruses, and in order to detect each virus' antigen, a different sample may be needed. Multiplex PCR assays and deep sequencing of CSF appear promising for improving the diagnosis.

On the other hand, encephalitis can be fatal and be linked to long-term consequences despite the fact that it frequently self-limits. The majority of viral meningitis cases are caused by enteroviruses, and many viral infections of the meninges and brain parenchyma can be avoided. Vaccination can reduce the spread of the tick-borne viruses that cause encephalitis, including the Japanese encephalitis virus.

Cerebrospinal Fluid Lactate

Cerebrospinal fluid lactate levels are significantly elevated in bacterial, as compared to viral meningitis and can provide pertinent, reliable, and rapid diagnostic information in differentiating bacterial from viral meningitis.

Chronic Meningitis

A clinical distinction between acute, subacute meningitis, and chronic meningitis is made based on an arbitrary time period of more than 4 weeks of symptoms and increasing CSF cell counts in chronic meningitis.

Identifying a cause for the chronic meningitis and providing appropriate treatment is a challenge, as many of the causative organisms are rare and the cause itself could be noninfectious. Medications, toxins, noninfective inflammatory conditions, and malignancies, and especially the autoimmune disorders can cause clinical features mimicking an infection.

A thorough history, evaluation of the clinical findings and epidemiological considerations, are needed for establishing the diagnosis. Numerous serological, CSF, and neuroimaging investigations are frequently necessary.

Numerous novel noninvasive diagnostic methods, including metagenomic deep sequencing, multiplex PCR, and 16s, 18s, and 28s, ribosomal RNA PCR, assist in identifying a wide variety of pathogens.

Chronic meningitis is most often indolent and is caused by rare and diverse infective agents, apart from a significant number being secondary to noninfectious agents. Treatment, which is often empirical will vary from case to case.

The most frequent fungus cause of chronic meningitis, *Cryptococcus neoformans*, still has a long-term death rate of at least 25%. Survival in cryptococcal meningitis is improved by rapid reduction of increased intracranial pressure. Repeated therapeutic lumbar punctures are helpful to decrease the pressure.

A number of viruses are implicated in causing chronic meningitis and meningoencephalitis namely HIV, *Cytomegalovirus* (CMV), HSV-1 and HSV-2, polyomavirus, enterovirus, lymphocytic choriomeningitis virus, and mumps virus.

Chronic meningitis in HIV-infected people is caused by tuberculous meningitis (TBM) and cryptococcal opportunistic infections, which might appear at the time of seroconversion.

Meningitis that is acute, chronic, or recurring is frequently brought on by HSV-2. Amongst the bacterial causes of chronic meningitis, *Mycobacterium tuberculosis* (MTB) and treponema pallidum are the important organisms responsible.

Chronic meningitis also occurs due to tick-borne organisms of *Ehrlichia*, *Babesia*, and *Anaplasma* species, as well as other bacteria such as *Nocardia*, *Leptospira*, *Brucella*, and *Listeria*.

Despite their rarity, parasite infections, which can be caused by organisms including *Echinococcus*, *Strongyloides*, *Acanthamoeba*, *Taenia solium*, and *Toxoplasma* species, should be taken into account while making a differential diagnosis. In our country, neurocysticercosis, malaria, and hydatidosis are widely prevalent.

A number of autoimmune inflammatory conditions can lead to a chronic meningitis state mimicking an infection. Immunoglobulin G4 (IgG4)-related neurological manifestations include pachymeningitis and pituitary gland involvement. The Vogt–Koyanagi–Harada syndrome involves the ocular system and the meninges, while sarcoidosis affects the cranial nerves, meninges, and the brain parenchyma apart from the spinal cord.

Metastasis of solid and hematologic malignancies, to leptomeningitis and pachymeninges, is also a cause of chronic meningitis. Carcinomatous meningitis can mimic an infectious meningitis, with an enhanced CSF cell count, low CSF to serum glucose, and elevated protein may be caused by the metastatic spread.

Cerebrospinal fluid cytology, flow cytometry immunophenotyping and meningeal biopsy may be required to identify the spread from breast and lung cancer, melanoma, lymphoma, and leukemia to involve the meninges.

Differential Diagnosis of Parenchymal Enhancement on MRI

Infections
- Acute bacterial meningitis
- Mycobacterial TB
- Viral (HTLV-1 and herpes virus)
- Fungal (*Cryptococcus* and *Coccidioides*)
- Syphilis and amoebic

Autoimmune Disorders
- Sarcoid
- IgG4-related meningeal involvement
- Rheumatoid arthritis (RA) and Sjogren syndrome
- Vogt–Koyanagi–Harada syndrome
- Granulomatosis

Neoplasms
- Metastasis from breast, lung, and melanoma
- Focal enhancement of meningioma
- Glioneuronal tumor

Iatrogenic Causes
Lumboperitoneal shunt, intrathecal chemotherapy, and craniotomy.

Other Causes
- Cerebral venous sinus thrombosis (CVST)
- Spontaneous intracranial hypotension (SICH)
- Post SAH (subarachnoid hemorrhage)
- Extramedullary hematopoiesis
- Idiopathic cause

Differential Diagnosis of Leptomeningeal (Pia Arachnoid) Enhancement on Magnetic Resonance Imaging
- *Infections*:
    - Acute pyogenic meningitis
    - Viral
- *Predominant basal enhancement* in TBM, listeria, fungi, *Amoeba*, and syphilis
- *Autoimmune disorders*—sarcoid, histiocytosis, Behcet's, IgG4, Vogt-Koyanagi-Harada syndrome
- *Neoplasm*—diffuse leptomeningeal glioneuronal tumor, leptomeningeal carcinomatosis, and lymphoma

TUBERCULOSIS OF THE CENTRAL NERVOUS SYSTEM

Fever, vomiting, headaches, and apathy are among the symptoms of TBM. Cranial nerves do get affected quite often, as there is basal meningitis and involvement of the ambient cistern through which the nerves pass. The 2nd, 3rd, 7th, 6th, and 8th cranial nerves are most often involved. Imaging could reveal enhancement of basal meninges, dilatation of the ventricles, and infarctions in the supratentorial and brainstem regions.

Hyponatremia does occur in almost half of the patients with TBM, and should be looked for and treated. It is most frequently due to cerebral salt wasting.

Although the CSF in TBM exhibits a modest pleocytosis comparable to that seen in viral or fungi infections, the quantity of protein is higher than it is in most other types of CNS infections. A cobweb is formed by the protein if allowed to stand for >12 hours. The cells seen are lymphocytes but in the early phases, polymorphs could predominate.

Cerebrospinal fluid culture for *MTB* takes 2-4 weeks to become positive and hence treatment should be started on an empiric basis at the earliest. Acid fast bacilli are difficult to be found on Ziehl-Neelsen stain, even by an experienced technician.

The sensitivity of smear and culture are 37% and 52%, respectively, when only one CSF examination is done while it increases to 87% and 83% if three samples are examined. Given that coinfection reduces both the sensitivity and specificity of TB tests, HIV status should be determined at the time of diagnosis.

Adenosine Deaminase

It is an enzyme involved in the metabolism of purines and is linked to lymphocyte proliferation and differentiation. Elevated levels signify generalized CNS injury and increased blood-brain barrier permeability. Most forms of meningitis are accompanied by elevated levels of adenosine deaminase (ADA) in the CSF, which are closely correlated to CSF protein levels.

Tuberculosis Polymerase Chain Reaction (PCR for MTB)

The PCR assays may be more sensitive than CSF cultures, but even a negative PCR result cannot rule out the diagnosis of TBM. The diagnostic criteria used, the amount of CSF taken, and whether anti-TB treatment (ATT) had previously been initiated all have a significant impact on the sensitivity and specificity of PCR assays for *MTB*.

Cartridge-based Nucleic Acid Amplification Test

The World Health Organization (WHO) has designated this test [Xpert MTB/resistance to rifampicin (RIF) assay], which can identify

MTB as well as mutations linked to rifampicin resistance, as the optimal initial test for TBM. The *LTA4H* gene has polymorphisms that affect the likelihood of inflammation in TBM has 100% sensitivity and specificity in tubercular meningitis.

Tuberculoma (Tuberculous Granuloma)

About 10% of persons with TBM also have tuberculomas and a third of them have multiple. This scenario is especially seen in children while on treatment for TBM. Tuberculomas without occurrence of TBM are quite common in our country. The clinical presentation consists of headache, seizures, focal neurological deficits, and papilledema.

The centers of tuberculomas caseate and liquefy, causing hypointense to isointense to hyperintense imaging characteristics on T2 and fluid-attenuated inversion recovery (FLAIR) MRI sequences. There is no pathognomonic neuroimaging characteristic for a tuberculoma of the brain **(Figs. 1A and B)**.

IMMUNE RECONSTITUTION INFLAMMATORY SYNDROME

This condition is an inflammatory reaction to an undiagnosed infection particularly HIV infection and after beginning highly active antiretroviral therapy (HAART). Immune reconstitution inflammatory syndrome (IRIS) can occur in the setting of a

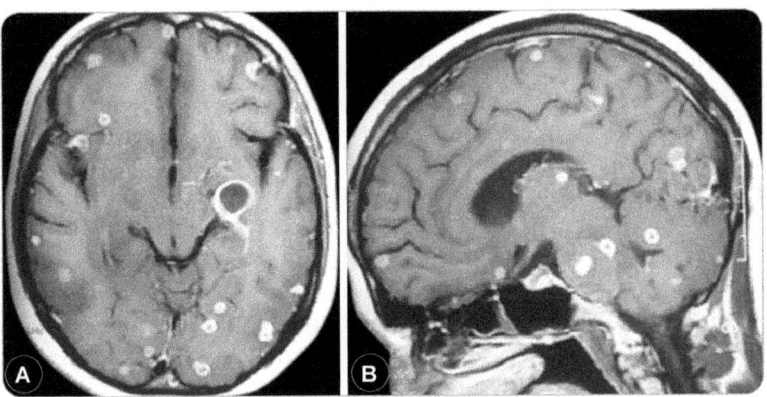

FIGS. 1A AND B: MRI brain T1 contrast axial and sagittal view showing multiple ring-enhancing conglomerate lesions suggestive of tuberculoma.

previously treated infection and with recovery through HAART treatment. This is called paradoxical IRIS.

Patients with a median CD4+ count of generally <50 cells/mm and a median of 4 weeks after beginning HAART are most likely to develop a mycobacteria infection associated with IRIS. It frequently presents with fever and the clinical worsening of pre-existing lymphadenopathy (in 70% of cases), respiratory distress (30% of the time), or CNS symptoms.

TREATMENT OF CENTRAL NERVOUS SYSTEM TUBERCULOSIS

For TBM, the WHO advises taking the same drug regimen as for pulmonary TB, 10 months of rifampicin and isoniazid followed by 2 months of rifampicin, isoniazid, pyrazinamide, and ethambutol (WHO guidelines for treatment of drug susceptible TB and patient care. Published April 2017).

Based on the presence of HIV and the assumed susceptibility of the TB organism, empiric treatment should begin as soon as CNS TB is suspected rather than waiting for confirmation. The two antibacterial drugs isoniazid and pyrazinamide had the best subarachnoid space penetration.

TUBERCULOSIS RESISTANCE

Drug resistance makes treating all types of TB more difficult. Drug resistance typically arises when a patient who was sensitive does not complete the required course of treatment, does not follow it strictly, or takes inappropriate treatment. Additionally, drug resistance can be passed on, which is where pharmacogenomics will be helpful.

Mycobacterium tuberculosis that is resistant to isoniazid and rifampicin is referred to be multidrug-resistant TB.

If MTB is resistant to isoniazid, rifampicin, a quinolone antibiotic, and one of the second-line injectables such as kanamycin, capreomycin, and amikacin, it is said to have extensive multidrug resistance. WHO advises that all patients with severe or multidrug-resistant TB follow a directly observed treatment plan (DOTS) in addition to receiving a second-line anti-TB medicine.

Corticosteroids use in TBM, as a concomitant treatment agent, is recommended and is being increasingly used. Administration of corticosteroids decreases mortality in TBM, at least in the short term, according to a meta-analysis of seven RCTs comparing ATT with or without them.

For all TBM patients, the WHO advises starting adjuvant corticosteroid therapy with dexamethasone or prednisolone and tapering it over 6–8 weeks. The most popular dosage for dexamethasone is 12–16 mg/day for 3 weeks, followed by a 3-week taper. If more time is needed, the tapering process can be prolonged, and if the situation gets worse, the dose can be raised.

Follow-up neuroimaging on patients with TBM has shown that patients who received dexamethasone had fewer complications of cerebral infarction and hydrocephalus.

HERPES SIMPLEX VIRUS ENCEPHALITIS

Herpes simplex virus-1 causes encephalitis and HSV-2 causes meningitis though encephalitis can also occur. HSV encephalitis either due to HSV-1 or HSV 2, is one of the most devastating encephalitides. Although the pathophysiology is unclear, it comes from the reactivation of latent illness and intraneuronal virus propagation into the brain parenchyma. HSV encephalitis carries a mortality of up to 70% when not treated and even when treated, only a little over a third return to normality.

The clinical features associated with HSV encephalitis include seizures in about 30%, abnormal behavior in 25%, loss of consciousness and confusion or disorientation in about 12%. Fever, autonomic dysfunction, and dysphagia are common presenting features.

The most frequent cause of treatment delays, which are linked to increased morbidity and death, is failing to include HSV in the differential diagnosis at an early stage.

Cerebrospinal fluid must be examined for cell count, biochemistry, and viral DNA using PCR for the diagnosis. The sensitivity and specificity of the HSV PCR are 96% and 99%, respectively. Based on the results of the CSF study, it is recommended to rule out additional diagnostic possibilities such bacterial and fungal meningitis.

White blood cell counts in the CSF were normal in about one-fourth of HSV encephalitis patients. If the clinical suspicion is high and the initial testing was negative, the treatment should be continued and the HSV PCR should be redone in 3–7 days.

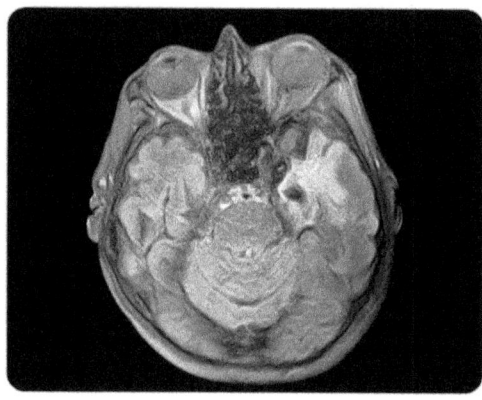

FIG. 2: Axial fluid-attenuated inversion recovery magnetic resonance imaging brain showing left temporal lobe hyperintensity as seen in herpes simplex encephalitis.

Hemorrhagic necrosis and edema in the medial temporal lobes are caused by HSV encephalitis, which can also affect limbic regions, the insula, cingulate, and inferolateral frontal cortices. By displaying distinctive medial temporal lobe imaging findings, MRI can help with the diagnosis **(Fig. 2)**.

Many times, both acute and chronic HSV encephalitis are accompanied by seizures. Refractory status epilepticus, which can have devastating sequelae and difficult to treat, is frequently the outcome of intractable seizures.

Treatment

Acyclovir intravenous infusion is essential for lowering HSV infection-related morbidity and mortality. 10 mg/kg IV every 8 hours for 14–21 days is the suggested dosage. Foscarnet should be tested when acyclovir resistance is detected as a result of clinical deterioration. Even while there is evidence of benefit, particularly in individuals with cerebral edema, the use of steroids in HSV encephalitis is still debatable, according to the literature.

About 2–6 weeks following HSV encephalitis, about 20% of individuals may go on to develop an autoimmune encephalitis with antibodies to the N-methyl-D-aspartate (NMDA) receptor.

CHAPTER 13

Dementia

INTRODUCTION

Dementia is a condition in which memory, thinking, and social abilities are affected with significantly enough to interfere with activities of daily life. Memory impairment is an important and common component of dementia, but memory impairment alone does not constitute dementia, though it would qualify for minimal cognitive impairment (MCI).

COGNITIVE IMPAIRMENT

Cognitive impairment can be minimal, called minimal cognitive impairment (MCI), when cognitive involvement is only in one domain; or can be major neurocognitive impairment when there is involvement in more than one domain and is considered dementia when it interferes with social activities and functioning.

Memory involvement is, however, not a must in either of these conditions though, however, it is the predominant domain affected in both.

The symptoms suggesting dementia are:
- Memory loss noted by a family member
- Difficulty in communicating
- Difficulty in navigating the way and getting lost while walking or driving

- Difficulty with reasoning or problem solving
- Difficulty in handling complex tasks

Psychological changes may be associated with the cognitive changes and these include:
- Personality changes
- Depression
- Anxiety
- Inappropriate behavior
- Paranoia
- Agitation
- Hallucination

CAUSES OF DEMENTIA

These include reversible causes and irreversible causes, which result in a progressive major cognitive disorder.

Causes of dementia syndrome and dementia-like symptoms which reverse with treatment are:
- Encephalopathies which include infections and immune-mediated disorders
- Metabolic derangements and endocrinopathies such as hypothyroidism, neuroglycopenia, hyponatremia, and hypocalcemia.
- Nutritional deficiencies due to vitamin B1, B6, B12 deficiencies, copper, vitamin D, and vitamin E deficiency
- Dehydration-related encephalopathy
- Adverse effects of medications especially anticholinergics, and interaction of several medications
- Subdural hematomas (SDH) where dementia-like symptoms are a common presenting feature.
- Poisoning and toxins exposure such as lead, pesticide exposure, and consumption of recreational drugs and excess of alcohol.
- Brain tumors especially frontal lobe tumors
- Normal pressure hydrocephalus (NPH)
- Hypoxic encephalopathy

All of the above could occur as acute, subacute, or chronic encephalopathies with cognitive involvement, thereby simulating dementing illness but are reversible with treatment to a variable extent.

RISK FACTORS

The risk factors which contribute to dementia include those which cannot be changed and those which can be changed.

Risk Factors that cannot be Changed
- *Age*: Risk rises with age over 65 years though dementia is not a normal accompaniment of aging.
- *Family history*: Those with a family history of dementia have a greater risk, though many in the family might not have lived long enough to have had dementia when they were alive.
- *Down's syndrome*: Many persons with Down's syndrome tend to develop early-onset Alzheimer's disease (AD).

Risk Factors that can be Changed
Diet and Exercise
Lack of exercise increases the risk of dementia. Research indicates a greater risk of dementia in those whose diet differs from Mediterranean style diet which is rich in whole grains, nuts, and seeds. Heavy alcohol use, i.e., large amounts of alcohol daily, increases the risk of dementia. Cardiovascular risk factors for dementia include high cholesterol levels, atherosclerosis, and obesity. Diabetes is a risk factor, especially when it is poorly controlled. Sleep apnea, if not corrected, could lead to cognitive impairment. Vitamin and nutritional deficiency of vitamin D, vitamin B1, B6, B12, and folate can cause cognitive deficits.

Problems Associated with being Demented
- Poor nutrition, as their intake becomes progressively less.
- Pneumonia, secondary to aspiration due to swallowing difficulty.
- Poor selfcare, needing assistance, or becoming dependent for activities of daily living (ADL) on others.
- Having personal safety issues.

SLOWLY PROGRESSIVE DEMENTIAS

The most prevalent kind of progressive dementia in the world is Alzheimer's disease (AD). Memory impairment is one of the early and key features followed by word-finding difficulty and anomia.

Diagnostic Criteria for Alzheimer's Disease

Multiple cognitive deficits manifested by:
- Impairment of memory (amnesia)
- Aphasia
- Apraxia
- Agnosia and
- Disturbance in executive functioning

The cognitive deficits should be significant enough to cause impairment in occupational and social functioning, and the impairment should be progressive. Most cases are sporadic with about 5% of persons having an autosomal dominant inheritance of mutations in the gene *presenilin 2 (PS2), amyloid precursor protein (APP)* and *presenilin1 (PS1)*. Presence of amyloid neuritic plaque and neurofibrillary tangles is the pathological hallmark features of AD.

- *Magnetic resonance imaging (MRI)* shows no specific changes in AD and is usually normal in the early stages. In the later stages, atrophy of hippocampus and cortex becomes apparent **(Figs. 1A and B)**.
- *Positron emission tomography (PET) scan* shows hypometabolism in temporal and parietal cortex. Raised tau protein with decreased Aβ42 amyloid and increased ceramide levels in cerebrospinal fluid (CSF) are recognized biomarkers.

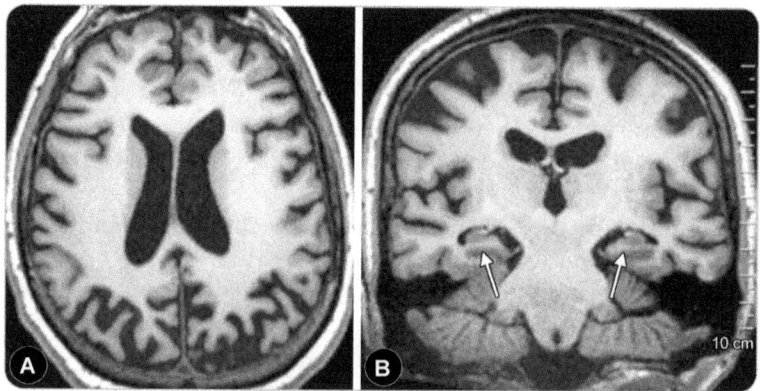

FIGS. 1A AND B: (A) Cortical atrophy in fluid-attenuated inversion recovery (FLAIR) axial magnetic resonance imaging (MRI) brain and (B) bilateral hippocampal atrophy (white arrows).

Treatment

Central cholinesterase inhibitors are used and these include:
- Donepezil with a long half-life
- Rivastigmine is also available in a patch form, with a long duration of action.
- N-methyl-D-aspartate (NMDA) glutamate antagonist, memantine, helpful in early and moderately severe cases
- Aducanumab, a monoclonal antibody, which targets amyloid protein and removes the plaque, is yet to be used on a mass scale, and early results are not impressive.
- LECANEMAB is the recent more promising monoclonal antibody but more strides are needed.

VASCULAR DEMENTIA

Perhaps the second most common form of dementia in our country is *vascular dementia (VaD)*.

Dementia can occur with vascular lesions in the following situations:
- Multiple infarcts involving both hemispheres.
- Diffuse white matter ischemic changes because of small vessels involvement **(Fig. 2)**
- Infarct in a strategic area, like the thalamus **(Figs. 3A and B)**

Multi-infarct dementia can occur as a result of large infarcts or multiple bilateral small infarcts. Diffuse white matter involvement can also cause subcortical dementia.

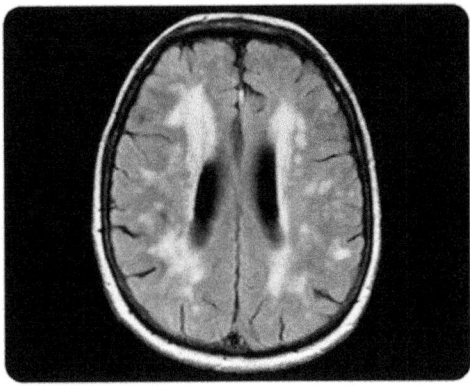

FIG. 2: Diffuse periventricular white matter changes along with multiple infarcts in fluid-attenuated inversion recovery (FLAIR) axial magnetic resonance imaging (MRI) brain.

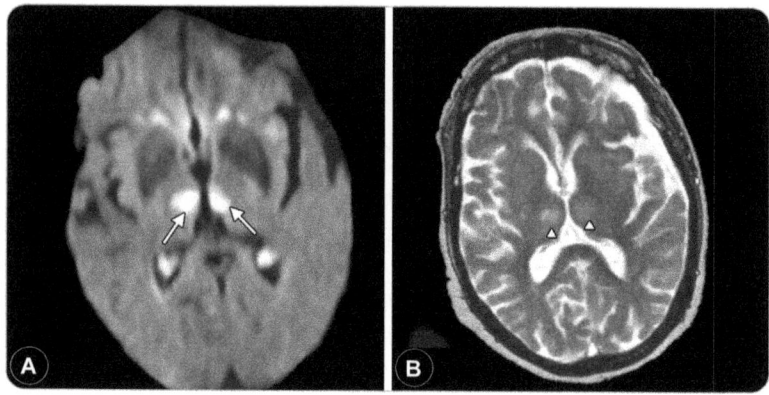

FIGS. 3A AND B: Acute diffusion restriction lesion in bilateral thalamus (strategic infarct) and T2 hyperintensity in the same region in T2 axial magnetic resonance imaging (MRI) brain.

FRONTOTEMPORAL DEMENTIA

Frontotemporal dementia (FTD) is the second common *degenerative* dementia with features of:
- Decline in personal hygiene
- Lack of awareness, and abnormal behavior and thought
- Changes in food preferences like craving for sweet, and consumption of inedible objects
- *C9ORF72* expanded mutations of FTD, can present with features of visual and auditory hallucinations.

Speech and Language Problems in Frontotemporal Dementia

Two types of primary progressive aphasias (PPA) are considered to be manifestations of FTD and these are characterized by increasing difficulty in using and understanding written and spoken language.

Semantic dementia is one, wherein individuals have prominent difficulty with naming (anomia) and replace a specific word with a more general word such as "it", for pen, and also lose the knowledge of the meaning of the word, which is the hallmark of this semantic type. Another type of PPA is progressive agrammatic aphasia, characterized by hesitancy in speech which becomes telegraphic with misuse of pronouns and errors in sentence construction resembling nonfluent dysphasia. The progressive nature distinguishes the acute nonprogressive aphasias from these types of FTD.

Movement Disorders in Frontotemporal Dementia

Some subtypes of FTDs are associated with movement-related issues such as tremor, rigidity, muscle spasms, incoordination, muscle weakness, and difficulty in swallowing.

Several Clinical Subtypes of Frontotemporal Dementia

- Behavioral variant FTD (bvFTD)
- Semantic variant PPA (svPPA)
- Nonfluent/agrammatic variant PPA (nfvPPA)
- Logopenic variant PPA (lvPPA)
- FTD-associated motor neuron disease (MND) (FTD-MND)
- FTD-associated corticobasal syndrome (CBS) (FTLD TDP-43)
- FTD-associated progressive supranuclear palsy (PSP) (FTLD-tau)

The last two (CBS and PSP) are tau-associated neurodegenerative disorders which can present with frontal lobe dysfunction and are referred to as FTD-related disorders.

The clinical subtypes of FTD and related disorders are defined based on the of symptoms and signs observed, and the variations in clinical presentation across the subtypes these are attributed to involvement of different brain regions by the FTD pathology.

The term frontotemporal lobar degeneration (FTLD) is reserved for patients with clinical presentations of FTD and identification of an FTD causing mutation or histopathologic evidence of FTD (on biopsy or postmortem).

Approximately 40% of FTD is associated with an AD pattern of inheritance. bvFTD and nfvPPA are common phenotypes of genetic FTD. Mutations in approximately eight genes have been linked to FTD with mutations in *granulin (GRN)*, C9ORF72, and *microtubule-associated protein tau (MAPT)* accounting for the majority.

Neuropathology

Abnormal accumulations of tau or TAR DNA-binding protein 43 (TDP-43) account for the majority of pathologically confirmed cases of FTD, followed by fused in sarcoma (FUS) inclusions type

FTD. Tau inclusions are rare in semantic variant PPA which is almost always sporadic. TDP-43 pathology is found in patients with semantic variant PPA, FTD-MND, and bvFTD as well as in *C9ORF72*, *GRN*, and *valosin-containing protein (VCP)* mutation genetic variants.

Mutations in the FUS gene and the FUS pathology are associated with an earlier age of onset of FTD with prominent neuropsychiatric features and a more rapid course. Atrophy of the dominant anterior temporal pole is the characteristic finding in semantic variant PPA.

Diagnosis

No single test can identify FTD and the diagnosis will have to depend on identifying certain key clinical features with the exclusion of other causes. It can be quite challenging to diagnose FTD in the early stages, as symptoms often overlap with other conditions which involve the frontal lobe and also with psychiatric disorders with which it is often confused.

Imaging is mainly useful to exclude other conditions which have structural abnormalities **(Figs. 4A to F)**.

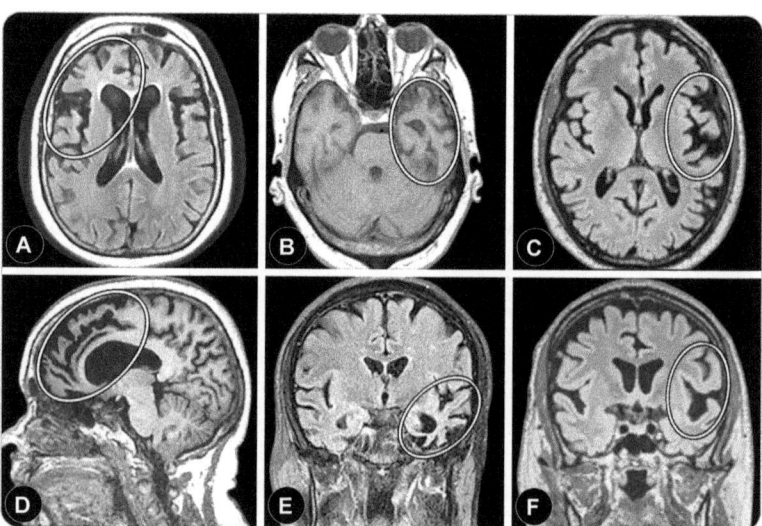

FIGS. 4A TO F: Magnetic resonance imaging brain showing anterior temporal atrophy and widened sylvian fissure as seen in typical frontotemporal dementia.

Fluorodeoxyglucose (FDG)—PET scan shows hypometabolism of frontal and temporal regions with left temporal polar atrophy in semantic variant of PPA. Pittsburg compound B (Pi B)—PET imaging or CSF Aβ1 to 42 and tau analysis helps differentiate FTD from frontal or language variants of AD. Options for pharmacotherapy are limited. Open label studies show no clear symptomatic benefit for cholinesterase inhibitors or memantine. Selective serotonin reuptake inhibitors (SSRIs) may modulate intrusive and compulsive behaviors in some patients.

DEMENTIA WITH LEWY BODIES

Dementia with Lewy bodies (DLB) is a type of dementia accompanied by changes in behavior, cognition, and movement.

It is a progressive disease with cognitive decline interfering with normal daily functioning.

- Rapid eye movement (REM) sleep behavior disorder (RBD) is a disorder in which persons lose the normal muscle paralysis occurring during REM sleep and act out their dreams as a core feature.
- Other frequent symptoms include, visual hallucinations, fluctuation in attention, and slowness of movement or rigidity.
- The autonomic nervous system is usually affected resulting in changes in blood pressure, heart, and gastrointestinal functions with constipation being a common symptom.
- Mood changes such as depression and apathy are common.

The DLB is one of the common types of dementia along with AD, FTD, and VaD. Together with Parkinson's disease dementia (PDD), it is one of the two dementias classified as Lewy body dementias (LBD).

$$DLB + PDD = LBD$$

Pathology

There is widespread deposits of abnormal clumps of alpha-synuclein protein and it is an alpha-synucleinopathy along with Parkinson's disease and multiple system atrophy (MSA). Treatment is essentially symptomatic and is oriented toward reducing the burden on the caregiver, as is being done with other dementias.

Acetylcholinesterase inhibitors such as donepezil and rivastigmine improve cognition and mental functioning, while melatonin helps sleep-related functioning. Antipsychotics are better avoided as patients with DLB are sensitive to these medicines and show worsening. This worsening with antipsychotics could serve as a diagnostic feature.

Diagnosis

The four core clinical features of DLB are:
1. Fluctuating cognition or attention
2. Visual hallucinations
3. REM sleep behavior disorder
4. Signs of Parkinsonism

The following serve as diagnostic findings of DLB:
- Decreased dopamine transporter uptake in the basal ganglia on PET/single photon emission computed tomography (SPECT) imaging
- Low uptake of iodine-metaiodobenzylguanidine (I^{123}-MIBG) seen on myocardial scintigraphy.
- Loss of atonia during REM sleep evidences on polysomnography

Symptoms Correlation with Sites of Involvement

Correlation of the areas of the brain involved with the various symptom complex affected in dementia.
- Cerebral cortex—thought, perception, and language
- Limbic cortex—emotions and behavior
- Hippocampus—memory
- Midbrain and substantia nigra—movement disorder
- Brainstem—sleep, alertness, and autonomic dysfunction
- Hypothalamus—autonomic dysfunction
- Olfactory cortex—smell
- Spinal cord and peripheral nervous system—autonomic dysfunction

HUNTINGTON'S DISEASE

Huntington's disease (HD) is an AD degenerative brain disorder. The characteristic features of the disease are chorea, cognitive disturbance, and psychiatric symptoms with age of onset in the fourth or fifth decade **(Fig. 5)**.

The disease affects the striatum predominantly with atrophy of the caudate nuclei visualized on neuroimaging studies, and

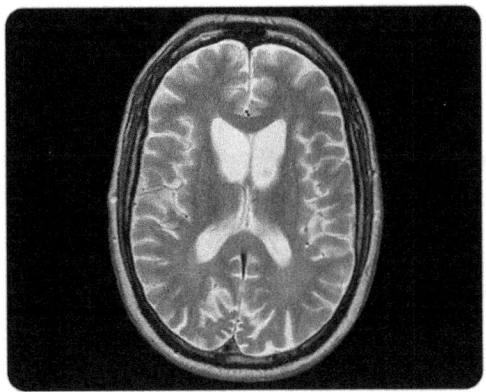

FIG. 5: Magnetic resonance imaging T2 axial brain showing bilateral head of caudate atrophy in Huntington's disease.

the disease results from impaired signaling from the cortex to the striatum. The HD gene is located on chromosome 4p containing a CAG trinucleotide repeat expansion and codes for a protein called Huntingtin.

Persons having >36 CAG repeats in the HD gene are likely to develop the disease if they live up to an advanced age and those having >40 CAG repeats develop the disease in the fourth or fifth decade itself. Huntington disease-like 2 (HDL-2) patients have a CTG repeat in *junctophilin 3 (JPH3)* gene.

PROTEINOPATHIES

The various proteinopathies associated with neurodegenerative disorders can be classified as:

Tauopathies:
- AD
- FTD
- CBD
- PSP

Synucleinopathies:
- Idiopathic Parkinson's disease (IPD)
- MSA
- DLBD

TDP-43 proteinopathies:
- Amyotrophic lateral sclerosis (ALS)
- FTD

RAPIDLY PROGRESSIVE DEMENTIAS

Dementias that progress rapidly are:
- Creutzfeldt–Jacob disease (CJD)
- Autoimmune encephalitis
- Central nervous system (CNS) vasculitis
- Infections such as herpes simplex virus (HSV) and human immunodeficiency virus (HIV)
- Progressive multifocal leukoencephalopathy (PML)
- Subacute sclerosing panencephalitis (SSPE)

Creutzfeldt–Jacob Disease

It is a fatal degenerative disorder with issues relating to memory and behavior associated with poor coordination and visual disturbances as early features, and later characterized by dementia, involuntary movements especially myoclonus, blindness, and weakness, progressing to coma.

About 70% die within a year of diagnosis. CJD is caused by a protein known as prion and hence referred to as prion disease. Infectious prions are misfolded prions that can cause normally folded proteins to become misfolded and lose function.

A small proportion (<8%) can occur as an AD inherited disorder. The differential diagnosis would be chronic meningitis or encephalitis. Onset is around 60 years of age and is classified as a type of transmissible spongiform encephalopathy (TSE). CJD is different from bovine spongiform encephalopathy (BSE) (mad cow disease), and variant CJD (vCJD). The misfolded prions affect signaling processes and damage the neurons resulting in degeneration, which causes the spongiform appearance in the affected brain.

Diagnosis is challenging, as in the early phase, the symptoms are nonspecific and the supportive diagnostic testing would include:
- Electroencephalogram (EEG) which may show specific periodic sharp wave complex discharges in about 50% of the people.
- Elevated levels of 14-3-3 protein in the CSF, considered to be supportive but not necessarily diagnostic.
- The real-time quaking-induced conversion (RT-QuIC) assay which has a diagnostic sensitivity of >80% and a specificity

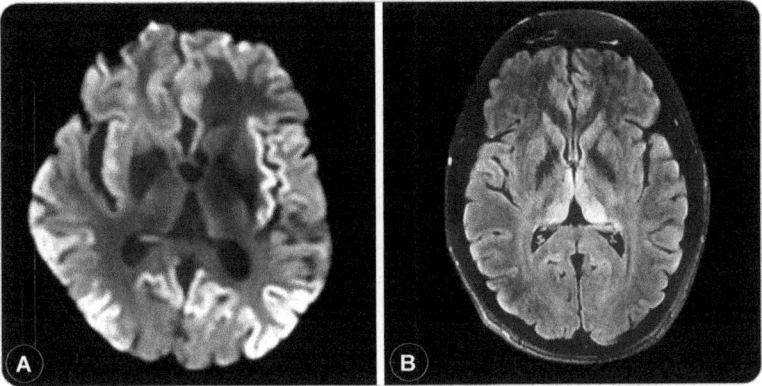

FIGS. 6A AND B: Magnetic resonance imaging (MRI) diffusion-weighted imaging shows cortical ribboning and bilateral thalamic fluid-attenuated inversion recovery (FLAIR) hyperintensity respectively, suggestive of Creutzfeldt–Jacob disease (CJD).

approaching 100% in CSF samples of patients with CJD. It has a high diagnostic value.
- The tumor marker, neuron-specific enolase (NSE) is often elevated in CJD and the diagnostic utility is increased when combined with an elevated 14-3-3 protein in CSF. MRI of the brain often shows high signal intensity in the caudate nucleus and putamen (striatum).
- Diffusion-weighted MRI sequences are the most sensitive and the characteristic features are focal or diffuse, diffusion restriction of the cerebral cortex and/or basal ganglia.

"Cortical ribboning" or "cortical ribbon sign" due to hyperintensities resembling ribbons appearing on the cortex on MRI is considered to be an iconic abnormality. The thalamus can be involved in the sporadic form and is seen more constantly in vCJD **(Figs. 6A and B)**.

Histopathological Examination

Tissue diagnosis remains the most definitive way of confirming the diagnosis of CJD, though it should be recognized that even biopsy is not always conclusive.

In 30% of sporadic CJD, prion protein scrapie Pr P^{sc} deposits are found in the skeletal muscle and/or the spleen.

Diagnosis of vCJD is supported by biopsy of the tonsils.

Biopsy of brain tissue is the definitive diagnostic test but a negative biopsy does not rule out CJD as it may predominate in a specific part of the brain which may not have been accessed on the biopsy.

Acquired Creutzfeldt–Jacob Disease

It is caused by contamination with tissue from an infected person and is usually iatrogenic. The medical procedures associated with transmission of CJD include:
- Blood transfusion from an infected person
- Human derived pituitary growth hormone injection
- Gonadotrophin hormone therapy
- Corneal and meningeal transplants from infected person

Variant Creutzfeldt–Jakob Disease

It is a type of acquired CJD, acquired from BSE in animals, by taking prion contaminated food. vCJD is one of the types of TSE.

In this condition, the symptoms are predominantly psychiatric with behavioral changes and painful sensations. Incubation period in believed to be in years and life expectancy is around a year after onset of symptoms. Though infection is primarily due to eating BSE-infected beef, a genetic susceptibility also exists. It is different from classic CJD, though both are due to prions.

The diagnosis can be suspected based on clinical features mentioned below, and brain biopsy is confirmatory:
- Mean age of onset is 28 years
- Mean duration varies from 13 to 14 months.
- Clinical signs and symptoms are psychiatric and behavioral, with dysesthesia and neurologic signs such as myoclonus, chorea, and hyperreflexia.
- Periodic sharp waves on EEG are often absent in vCJD.
- Caudate nucleus and putamen hyperintensity in FLAIR MRI is often absent.
- Pulvinar sign is seen as bilateral hyperintensities on axial FLAIR MRI in the pulvinar nuclei of the thalamus which resembles a reverse hockey stick and is pathognomonic and said to be present in about 75% of vCJD cases **(Fig. 7)**.

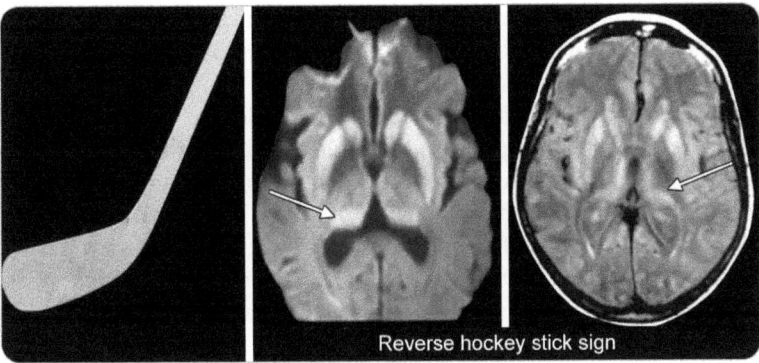

FIG. 7: MRI brain showing FLAIR hyperintensities in pulvinar region of the thalamus resembling reverse hockey stick in vCJD.

Autoimmune Encephalopathy and Dementia

This type of encephalopathy can be caused by a number of autoimmune disorders such as:
- Rasmussen encephalitis
- Systemic lupus erythematosus
- Behçet's disease
- Hashimoto's encephalopathy
- Autoimmune encephalitides

Immune-mediated cognitive deficits may result from *autoimmune dementia and encephalopathies (ADE)*. Presentations range from acute limbic encephalitis to chronic or subacute cognitive impairments that resemble neurodegenerative dementias. It might manifest as an idiopathic autoimmune phenomena or as a paraneoplastic syndrome. The clues to the diagnosis are:
- Presence of autoimmunity in the person or the family
- Evidence of inflammation in the CSF
- Serologic evidence of autoimmunity-directed against neural or nonorgan-specific antigens
- Mesial temporal MRI abnormalities

Neural-specific autoantibodies, which are pathogenic and responsive to immunosuppressant treatment, can attach to antigens on the cell surface such as NMDA receptor autoantibodies.

T-cell depleting immunotherapies have varying degrees of success in treating antibodies that bind to intracellular antigens, such as antineuronal nuclear autoantibody type (ANNA1 or Anti-HU), which are a marker for a T-cell-mediated process. It is crucial to find cancer early and treat it if it exists.

When the diagnosis is unclear, high dosage corticosteroids are the initial treatment, and the therapeutic response may also serve as a diagnostic test. Maintenance immunotherapy is advised for people who are at risk of recurrence. The prognosis varies, although it is worse for paraneoplastic autoimmune dementing encephalopathies (ADE) with intracellular antigen-specific antibodies. Cell surface antibodies are NMDA receptor, AMPA receptor, gamma-aminobutyric acid B (GABA-B) receptor, and glycine receptor antibodies. *LGI1* and *CASPR2* are antisynaptic antibodies and antineuronal antibodies are *ANNA1 (Hu), ANNA2 (Ri), ANNA3, Purkinje cell cytoplasmic antibody type 2 (PCA-2)*, amphiphysin-IgG antibodies.

Antisynaptic antibodies are *LGI1* and *CASPR2*.

Antineuronal antibodies are *ANNA1 (Hu), ANNA2 (Ri), ANNA3, PCA-2*, and amphiphysin IgG antibodies.

Index

A

Agnosia 61
Alzheimer's disease 130
Amitriptyline 5
Anxiety 15
Apraxia 57
ASPECTS Score 73
Aura 5
Agrin 91
Acute inflammatory demyelinating polyneuropathy (AIDP) 36
Anterior ischemic optic neuropathy (AION) 45
Albumino cytological dissociation 36
Aphasia 40
Aprosexia 48
Atypical Parkinsonian disorder 100-108
Autoimmune myopathies 91, 92

B

Balint syndrome 60
Blepharospasm 107
Benign paroxysmal positional vertigo (BPPV) 11
Brain death 66

C

Camptocormia 107
Capsular warning syndrome 77
CBNAAT 122
Cerebral venous sinus thrombosis 78
Creutzfeldt-Jakob disease (CJD) 138

Cluster headache 6
Cognition 48
Color agnosia 61
Comprehensive stroke center 71
Corticobasal syndrome 103

D

DAT Scan 104
Deep brain stimulation (DBS) 99
Dejavu 23
Dementia 127-142
Dementia with Lewy bodies (DLB) 135
Diabetic neuropathy 36
Dihydroergotamine 6
Dix-Hallpike maneuver 11, 13
Dizziness 10
Drop attacks 24
Dysautonomia 16

E

Eaton-Lambert syndrome 27
Eclampsia 54
Epley's maneuver 13, 14

F

Flunarizine 5
Frontotemporal dementia (FTD) 132-135
Fragile X tremor ataxia syndrome (FXTAS) 107

G

Guillain-Barré syndrome (GBS) 36
Gerstmann syndrome 58
Go-No-Go test 54

H

Head impulse test (HIT) 11
Head impulse, nystagmus, test of skew (HINTS) 15
Head thrust test (HTT) 11, 12
Hyperkinesias 114
Huntington's disease (HD) 136

I

Intracerebral hemorrhage 75-77
Idiopathic intracranial hypertension (IIH) 8

J

Juvenile myoclonic epilepsy (JME) 22
Jamais vu 23

L

Loss of consciousness (LOC) 20
Locked-in syndrome 65
Lithium 7
Lamotrigine 7
Leprous neuropathy 36
Language 49-50

M

Migraine 1, 21
Myopathies 27-31
Myoglobinuria 32
Minimally conscious state 66
Myoclonus 107
Meningitis 117-120
Medication overuse headache 9
Migralepsy 9
Memory 50, 51
Morvan syndrome 83
Musk antibody 91
Multiple system atrophy (MSA) 101

N

Narcolepsy 20
Neuropathies 33-37
NOACs 79

O

Osmophobia 4
Optic ataxia 60
Oculomotor apraxia 60
Optic neuritis 44
Optic atrophy 45

P

Phonophobia 4
Photophobia 4
Paroxysmal hemicrania 7
Praxis 57
Prosopagnosia 61
Persistent vegetative state 66
Parakinesia 110
Pseudoathetosis 111
Pachymeningitis 120
Polyneuropathy, organomegal, endocrinopathy, monoclonal gammopathy syndrome (POEMS) 35
Parkinson's disease (PD) 95-99
Progressive supranuclear palsy (PSP) 101

R

Reversible cerebral vasoconstriction syndrome (RCVS) 9
Relative afferent pupillary defect (RAPD) 44

S

Sumatriptan 6
Short-lasting unilateral neuralgiform headache with conjunctival injection and tearing (SUNCT) 7
Selective serotonin reuptake inhibitors (SSRI) 16
Seizures 19
Syncope 20
Subarachnoid hemorrhage 74

T

Tension type headache 1
Topiramate 5
Trigeminal autonomic cephalgia 1, 6
Temporal arteritis 8
Thunderclap headache 9
Tenecteplase 72
Transient ischemic attack (TIA) 77
Tics 112

V

Vertigo 10, 11
Vestibular migraine 13
Vestibular neuritis 15
Video EEG 19
Visual agnosia 61
Vein of Labbe 79
Vein of Trolard 79
Vein of Galen 79
Vascular dementia 131
Variant CJD (vCJD) 140

EU GSPR Authorised Reprsentative
Logos Europe, 9 rue Nicolas Poussin
1700, La Rochelle, France
Phone: +33 (0) 6 67 93 73 78
E-mail: contact@logoseurope.eu

www.ingramcontent.com/pod-product-compliance
Ingram Content Group UK Ltd.
Pitfield, Milton Keynes, MK11 3LW, UK
UKHW021018270326
469420UK00007B/66